WHY WE LIKE
OUR HOME FOOD

WHY WE LIKE
OUR HOME FOOD

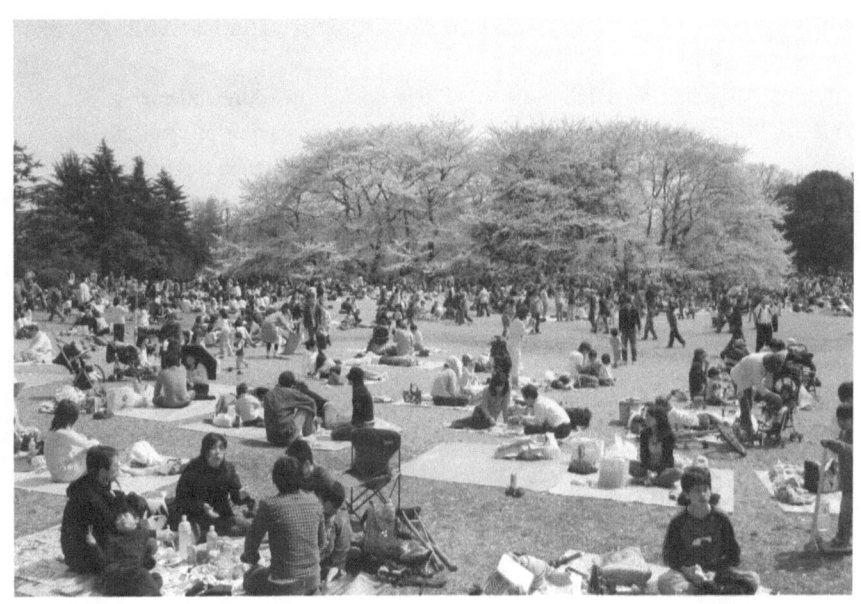

ALBERT YEUNG

To order additional copies of this book, contact:
Xlibris LLC
1-888-795-4274
www.Xlibris.com
Orders@Xlibris.com
616670

CONTENTS

Preface

This book is written for housewives, restaurant owners, and managers.

You can ask people what they like to eat in a social gathering. They may tell you they like their own home country's food. They may also tell you they have no idea or whatsoever. Now, you know how to plan the meal for them that they will like. You don't have to be a restaurant professional, and you can have more choices.

Like potluck with friends, everybody brings the food. It can be self prepared, or you buy it from restaurant. Comfort food like ice cream or soft food will be provided for those people who are sick or in a bad mood. The atmosphere is good. You can eat it in your own way. You can use hand or eat loudly. Nobody will stare at you. It can be table style or buffet style. You can watch TV as you are eating, or you are talking and eating at the same time. Those people you don't like, eg. those who are swearing when eating, can be asked to move to the other area. It is entertaining. You will remember it.

Meal planning is in our daily life. It is a good dining experience that make the meal great, no matter if it's for daily meals, social gatherings, or festival meals. For how many people do you have to prepare? How many courses? What do they like or dislike? Any precaution, like some having beef allergy? Happy or sad, just make some modifications. The price will be calculated every day to make sure it's affordable. Atmosphere is casual. You can eat last, finish your work first. If you don't like those social gatherings where you hear people asking when to make some money, when you will marry, you can take the food to the room to eat. It is happy. This pattern of eating life will last a long, long time. You will get used to it. It becomes part of your daily life.

The point behind this is the quality of food and the atmosphere. Food is always the first selection factor. Atmosphere, service, or price will be the second choice. When the other factors are not quite different, food will be the number one factor considered because it is our appetite that drives us to eat.

A good book means you like it. It may last a long, long time, like the Bible. The first thing is you like it. You feel happy when you read it. You can easily remember it or even apply the concept in your life. It may stay in your mind for a while, and you analyze the concept. You may keep it for reference. You take it out to check it, refine it, and apply it, like a recipe. It can function as a guideline for life.

It talks about enjoying the food in a professional manner. First, we talk about the food, the meal, the cooking, and the choice. Then, we talk about the enjoyment of the food. How is it served? How do you create the atmosphere so that it is entertaining and comfortable?

I find many people trying different ethnic foods, but finally they will still like their own home food. That's why I have the interest to find out the reason behind it. We understand the reason, then we can use the principle and apply it to enjoy the food.

It is hoped that you will like it. What you get is more than the cost of the book. Then, both of us will find it beneficial.

Introduction

Eating is a long history. Before we have written down any history of food, people ate raw food. The common one is eating animals they hunt, fish in the river, a pond, near seashore; and any wild fruit. Death rate was high due to issues on the sanitation and safety of food. Later, they learned to choose parts of the raw food. From experience, they knew which ones could be eaten and which ones were poisonous. Later, they found out that cooking food in fire is delicious. Fire could be caused by a storm and or the flashing of light. Then, they tried to make fire by themselves. Finally, they learned rubbing the branches of trees together. The friction could make fire. Cooking skill was improved by putting the animals, with their skin torn off, on the branch of a tree under the fire. This became a very popular way of outdoor cooking around the world, called barbecue. It has been more modified to cook with a large bowl with water. Cooking tools are used. Cooking is directly under fire. Then, salt becomes the seasoning.

Eating also changes from using hands to using tools. The introduction of forks and spoons completely changed the eating manners. With the advancement of science, we have canned and bottled drinks and packed food.

Ordinarily, we have the service of food. It is usually table service. It can be English, French, or Russian style. Family style is casual.

Food can be natural. Farming product began as people found it out by simply dropping some fruit seed into the cultivated land. Some products would grow by themselves. Nowadays, we choose the land and choose the farming products to grow. The product is also different in different parts of the world, according to climate and culture. Game animals are also raised in the farmland or in people's houses. Ranches are set up to raise horses, cattle, and sheep. Another product besides meat, feathers are also used for sale. Human-controlled "home fish, shrimps" are also found near the seashore.

The cooking and the tools are different. The common ones will be bowls, pans, cups. Cooking methods are steaming, frying, boiling. Seasoning is quite different, but the taste will be similar, whether salty, sweet, spicy. At restaurants, the cooking tools are different. They may be very large as a large volume of serving will be provided. The kinds of cooking tools are different and complicated to suit all kinds of cooking. The cooking method will be combined as more tools will be used.

The service will be more advanced. With fast service, the aim is to feed your stomach; convenience is the concept. Dinner is the enjoying time. Price is not important. Food and atmosphere are important. People go to a high class restaurant because they want to enjoy a good dinner. Of course, some go there to solve their life or job problems. It's a challenge to the hostess and the management. It may affect other customers. If the next table has people quarrelling and fighting or even talking, yelling, swearing loudly, the restaurant may have troubles.

People can watch a show, singing, or a dance while they have appetizers and refreshments. Fine food is then served. Social talking and eating go on the same time. Some may come here just for the food. Maybe they have a mini national feast that people want to try. There is good food, good service, and music is tender. It makes people enjoy a lot. The restaurant team will advise them on the wine-food pairing. They will be notified about any special event. Some good hotels are used by people for courting women.

The dining experience may still be on their minds even after they go home. That makes people go back again and again. It becomes their second home. It can be their second dining room or guest feast room. They like the service. Everything will be prepared for them.

Most of the time, a banquet is for social gathering or celebrating a famous event. A family meal is always the main focus of eating. At home, housewives have to meal-plan everything. They have to plan three meals. They have to decide the cost. How to cook it as different members may have eating preferences. Some like steaming while the others like frying. The atmosphere is good as the mother knows what they like to eat. They just decide sit on the table or watch the TV as they eat.

No matter what food material, cookware, or any cooking methods they use, how they enjoy it, what service manner it is, the dining experience you like is the most important thing. You will never refuse your home food.

Barbecue is an international dining experience. Each country, place, area may have little differences. It may be the tools, food, and cooking style. All know how to do it. Like our ancestors, they use fire to burn the food. Each one knows the culture to burn it, for example, praying before you cook. Marinate the meat, the hot dog, or prepare the salad. Imagine in the park or backyard, the smell of the meat cooking stimulates your appetite. Everyone cooks the food they like. You can cook for everybody or cook for yourself. You can cook again when you need more. The fire is easy to set as we have fast-burning charcoal or gas. You can sit aside to eat or to talk with your friends. At nighttime, you can have a campfire dance.

It's a nourishing of life. You will love your home food and the culture behind it. No matter if you are happy or sad, it can help you solve the problems.

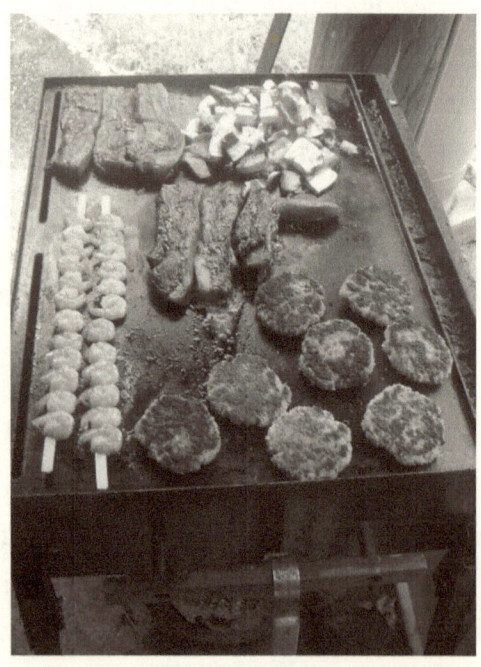

Food Quality

We prefer homeland food. Mother always makes the great food. She prepares, cooks, and eats in the way you like most. Don't forget, women are the natural good cooks. Again, it's a great dining experience that you can trust. After you try the famous food, New York steak, red wine, white wine, or a famous dinner, a banquet like the White House banquet, you still like your homeland food. You don't have to learn the etiquette, how to use the utensil, and learn how to eat the food. You don't feel embarrassed if the culture is different—for example, making noise when eating means you enjoy the food, but people in the US like to eat without noise. Each day, the mother plans the meal, what food to buy, how many to buy, which way to cook. When the meal is ready, you decide how to eat. Usually, it is free. You can eat in any way you like. Only in a formal dinner, you have to follow some etiquette. Only restaurants will have a menu study so that their food and service will attract more customers by competition.

A family cannot buy all the tools and materials like the big restaurant can. Housewives will buy what they can afford. The food materials are worldwide but different. Luckily, scientific developments can make the distance shorter so that you can buy everything without leaving your residence. Rice can be purchased anywhere in the world. Pizza can be made anywhere in the world too. The tools and materials can be imported. The materials can be in the form of frozen or fresh. Of course, people prefer fresh. Artificial food may lose its freshness. The cooking may be different as some areas prefer salty and sweet while the other areas like spicy. The gathering dinner may be for your family or include friends. The whole dining experience will be familiar.

Food must stimulate the appetite. It's the desire for food. The meaning of food means security, hospitality, and even status. Infants learn security when the mothers feed them when they are crying. Family food brings back memories of home, and family food makes one feel secure. Food is a way of hospitality and for friends to gather.

Flavor, texture, and appearance are the sensory characteristics of food. We judge the quality of food by our sensory evaluation. We eat and enjoy our food through our sense. Food may contain many flavor components that will impact the olfactory centers at different times. Thus, aroma, taste, and texture may change as we eat and drink. One good example is ice cream melting in the mouth.

There are several factors affecting the patterns of eating. The family structure and interactions among family members are important influences on the development of their food habits, their rigidity, and the ease at which they may be changed. It begins with infants but is modified as a child grows into adulthood and interacts with other people. Family meals play an important role in human communicating, for example, love, value, and information. The patterns of eating by individual and families are in a continuous process of change as their economic, social, and technical environments change.

Food behaviors are shaped by culture. Culture determines our food habits. Food patterns differ markedly from one culture to another. Within a culture, not everyone eats exactly the same. Individual preference may be different, and subgroups may develop. Families tend to develop their own distinctive food patterns, and individuals within a family have own personal food preferences. The ways they are different are not only in specific foods eaten, but also in the number of meals each day. Each culture passes on food habits and patterns by training children of which are acceptable or not, and patterns become familiar.

Sanitation and Safety

When dining out, we expect a clean facility, well-groomed workers, and a pleasant atmosphere. We also wish to have unseen sanitation and safety of food. They are regulated by laws and rules of food service. Managers and staff are expected to have safety certificates and food handling certificates. The management needs to train staff and arrange them to get a certificate. Policies are formulated, and rules are displayed at the right place.

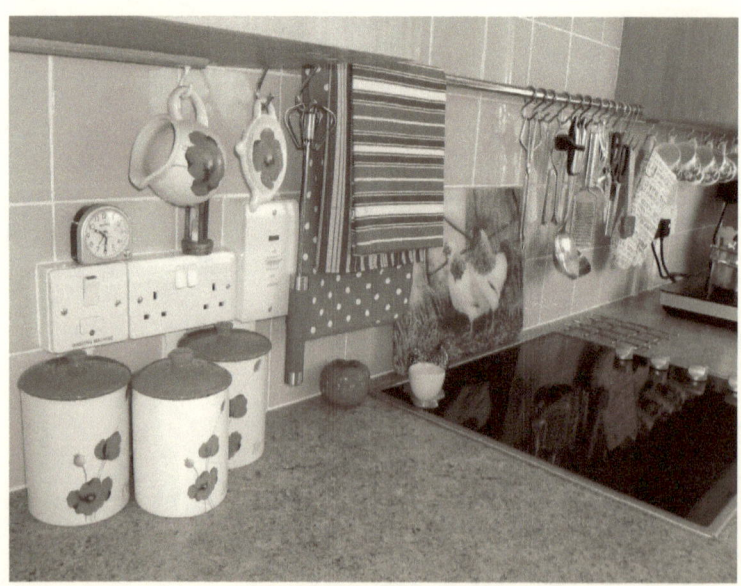

A safe food area means no slippery floor that may hurt people. A broken bowl or plate may hurt your mouth. A bended can of food may contaminate the food inside. It may also cut your fingers. Knives cannot be pointed at people. They have to point at the floor. Management must be knowledgeable and have a handbook of food code. Management must formulate the safety measures and monitor the staff and the area.

There are dangers of food-borne illness. It is the disease carried or transmitted to people by food. It may be due to cooking and holding food in the improper temperature. The staff must wash hands after going to the restroom for personal hygiene. The staff must be trained. A food safety system, HACCP, Hazard Analysis Critical Control Point, a food-safety management system, must be used by management. It's the prevention of food-borne illness by controlling hazards throughout the flow of food. It focuses on identifying specific points within the flow of food through the operation to prevent, eliminate, or reduce a biological, chemical, or physical hazard to safe levels. Those hazards are introduced by human or by the environment and naturally.

Microorganisms are responsible for the majority of food-borne illnesses. Microorganisms are small living creatures. Those that cause diseases are called pathogens. Eating food contaminated with pathogens or their toxins will cause food-borne diseases. There are four types of microorganisms that can contaminate food and cause food-borne diseases. They are bacteria, viruses, parasites, and fungi. They need food, acidity, temperature, time, oxygen, moisture to grow. So several way to prevent the growth of microorganisms are to add lactic acid to food; to add sugar, salt to lower its acidity; to move the food out of the temperature danger zone, 41°F to 135°F. It needs time to grow, so prepare it as soon as possible.

The measures to ensure food safety are controlling time and temperature, good personal hygiene, and cross-contamination. Microorganisms cannot survive outside certain temperature ranges. The range that bacteria grow in is called temperature danger zone. Personal hygiene is washing hands before and after handling food. Eating should be prohibited at the food preparation area or area for washing utensils. Sick staff will be excluded from the kitchen. Cross-contamination can be prevented by washing hands after working with raw food. Raw foods are not allowed to touch cooked food. Clean clothes between each use. Clean and sanitize the food contact surface.

The flow of food includes purchase and receiving. Choose an approved supplier and inspected food. The supplier should be reputable. The staff should be trained in the inspection of frozen food, fresh meat, eggs, fish, and vegetables. Meat and poultry should have a graded stamp by the USDA. They need to be at right temperature. Staff visual inspection will be used to sample-check the food. Any change of color or bad smell is a sign of bad food. A housewife can visually check or can ask the retailer about the freshness of the food.

Food will be stored at the right place and temperature. Rotate food products to ensure the oldest inventory is used first. Discard food that has passed the expiration date. Transfer foods between containers properly. Keep potentially hazardous food out of temperature danger zone. Check temperature of stored food and storage areas. Keep storage area clean. The housewife can put food in the refrigerator with meat at the bottom shelf. Food that can be stored longer can be put in the freezer.

The first thing in preparing food is to prevent contamination. Thaw food at refrigerators; use a clean work area, a clean cutting board, and a clean knife. Hands should be washed thoroughly. Remove food from refrigerator only in the amount needed. Cook as soon as possible. Check the cooked meat's internal temperature. Poultry is at 165°F; pork, beef, and lamb are at 145°F; fish is at 145°F; and egg is at 145°F. Food cooked below those temperatures are at the risk of introducing food-borne diseases.

Cooked food must be served immediately. Hot food that is held must have an internal temperature of 135°F. Food whose temperature is at the danger zone of 41°F to 135°F will be discarded. Replenish food on a timely basis. Keep raw meat, fish, and poultry separate from cooked and ready-to-eat food.

Clean all the service areas. Pests can carry and spread a variety of diseases. Develop and implement an integrated pest-management program. It can prevent pests from entering the establishment. Screen all windows and vents, install self-closing doors and air curtains. Fill or cover holes around pipes, and seal floors and walls. Pests are attracted to damp, dark, and dirty places. So dispose of garbage quickly and keep containers clean. Remove dirty dishes and uneaten food from tables, and clean them. Employing a licensed PCO to handle pest control is the overall measure.

The benefit of food safety includes helping to protect people from food-borne diseases. It can also preserve its quality. It will maintain the appearance, flavor, texture, consistency, and nutritional value of food. The last one is to lower the food cost due to the waste of food.

A family doesn't have training or requirement for food safety. It is by common sense and experience. There are labels of food storage, food handling, and food safety guidelines. It can be displayed at a public area, like a refrigerator. The family will train the basic rules of food safety to the children. It's a long history of food handling, including purchase, storage, preparation of food, cooking food, and service. It should be safe. Any announcement of food being unsafe and of poison must be noted, like the unhealthy, contaminated peanut butter. It should be discarded. For any food-borne disease that occurs, the cause and source must be found out. Measure must be taken to correct it.

Delicious

It is how you taste the food. Do you feel full, feel energetic, feel comfortable, and think it tastes good? You can eat them all and find them easily digested. It includes the appearance, smell, and taste. The good appearance, like color, can attract if you taste it. Smell can also be attractive. With some food, the smell can go around the whole house. Taste depends on how well-done the food is. It makes you easily to eat. Overcooking may cause a rubbery and tough taste. If seasoning is added, the amount is important. Overseasoning means you eat the seasoning only, not being able to savor the taste of food. It may also harm the health. A limited amount of seasoning is allowed, like with the salt. Going over the limit will cause high blood pressure.

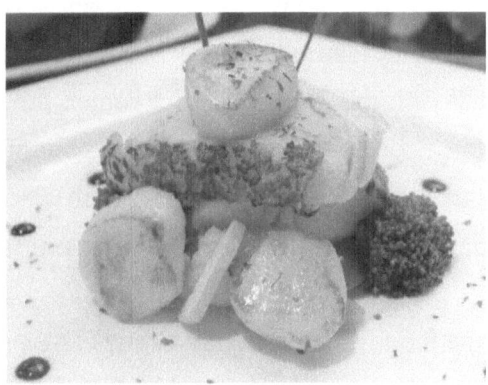

Appearance

It includes color, form, size and arrangement. Without an attractive appearance, the food may be rejected. The freshness of the food is also indicated by the smell of the food. For example the bad smell of meat means it is not consumable. It also indicates safety. Mold on fruit or vegetable means it should be discarded. Qualities of food are evaluated by the senses. Its being colorful means it is the first thing that you want to try. Nowadays, the appearance arrangement is more professional. Some make it like an art. The food can be made like an animal. Art is for you to like it but not for eating. So making it eatable is the main objective of appearance arrangement. Tomato soup looks like a flowing red liquid. It can stir your appetite. A whole ham that needs carving is more attractive than a piece.

Aromatic

Odor is a smell, pleasant or unpleasant, perceived through the stimulation of the olfactory center. The perceived flavor results from the integrated response to a complex stimuli from the olfactory centers in the nasal cavity, the taste buds on the tongue, tactile receptors in the mouth, and the perception of heat, coolness when a food is placed on the mouth. Flavor is a blending of taste and odor. Aroma is referred to as good odor. To stimulate our olfactory center, the substance must be in gaseous form. The gas enters the nose as we place food in the mouth and is drawn toward the olfactory center, where it stimulates the nerve endings. A neurotransmission is then sent to the brain.

You can smell the food when it is ready. Some can be smelled around the whole room. It is because hot oil and high temperature can cause the smell to spread. If the smell is good, it can stir your appetite.

Taste

Taste is the sensation perceived through the stimulation of taste buds on the tongue. The primary ones are sweet, salty, sour, and bitter. The sensations are produced through the stimulation of taste buds on the tongue. Taste buds are found in small elevations, the papillae, on the surface of tongue.

The physical properties of food include texture, consistency, and shape. It involves the sense of touch and feeling, called tactile taste. When food is touched, the tongue is stimulated. Sensation of smoothness, lumpiness will be detected. Moistness, dryness, hardness, or softness are the extreme conditions of texture. Sound is an enjoyment of food. Crispness or tenderness by the sound will be evaluated by the tactile sensation of the tongue. Then, we can decide the food is stale, musty, fragrant, spicy, fishy, or grassy.

After we feel the food is good or not, we begin to digest it. Well-done food will be delicious. Overcooked food may taste tough. Seasoning can also change the taste. Temperature is an important factor in determining the taste. Different temperatures may produce different tastes. Cold meat is not muscular and tender, but tough. It is also not safe to eat the food whose temperatures within the danger zone. It can be detected by its smell, color of food.

Conclusion

Food is delicious because of its appearance, smell, taste, or a combination of these three factors. Food is good, but before it enters your stomach, you need to watch the temperature. It may affect the food qualities. Temperature may affect the blending of the primary taste and other factors that determine flavor. Within the temperature range at which most foods are eaten, a temperature is marked in the intensity of the primary tastes. Food that is too hot may hurt the tongue. Food needs to be fully cooked to be safe. Undercooked food, like meat, may cause disease.

Nutrition

Nutrients are substances that are vital for the growth and maintenance of a healthy body throughout life. They come from food. There are six various classes of nutrients: carbohydrates, lipids, proteins, vitamins, minerals, and water. Food can provide energy, and it comes from carbohydrates, lipids, and proteins. Energy is expressed in terms of calories.

A basic plan for health promotion and disease prevention includes eating a varied diet, performing regular physical activity. The focus of nutrition planning should be on food. The focus on food to supply nutrient needs avoiding the possibilities of severe food imbalances. Avoid smoking, make sure you get adequate fluids and sleep, limit alcohol, and limit stress.

Recommendation for food choice can be by guidelines. A good menu planning tool is the food guide pyramids. It's a triangle of food that shows the hierarchy of food according to portions they should be served. The top is fats, oils and sweets. They are sparingly used. Next is the milk, yogurt, and cheese group. The other is meat, poultry, fish, dry beans, eggs, and nuts group. Both are given in two to three servings. The next is vegetable group. Another is the fruit group.

Both are two to four servings. The bottom of the pyramid is bread, cereal, rice, and pasta group and is six to eleven servings. This guide does not apply to infants or children under two years of age.

Carbohydrate is a primary source for some cells. Muscles rely on a supply of carbohydrates to support physical activity. The energy from carbohydrates per gram is four kilocalories. Fiber is an important class of carbohydrate. It provides health benefit. Food rich in carbohydrates are table sugar, honey, ham, jelly, fruit, and plain baked potatoes. An intake of fifty grams of carbohydrate per day is needed. But dietary fiber is twenty to thirty grams per day. Inadequate carbohydrate results in a loss of body protein, ketosis, and the weakening of the body.

Lipid contains more than twice the energy per gram, nine kilocalories, as protein and carbohydrates do. Lipids are relatively oxygen-poor compounds. They include saturated fatty acids, monounsaturated fatty acids, and polyunsaturated fatty acids. Cholesterol forms vital hormones. Foods rich in fat are salad oils, butter, margarine, and mayonnaise. It provides energy. It can also store energy. It insulates and protects our body organs, like the kidney. It can also transport fat-soluble vitamins. Fat should be 30 percent of total energy intake. Cholesterol intake will be limited to two hundred to three hundred milligrams per day. Deficiency in lipids will cause flaky skin, diarrhea, and infections.

Protein functions to regulate and maintain the body. The amino acid is the building block of protein. It determines the protein's ultimate shape and function. Proteins produce vital body constituents, maintain fluid balance, contribute to acid-base balance, form hormones, and provide energy. Protein-rich food includes water-packed tuna, beef, poultry, milk, bread, and cheese. We need 0.8 grams of protein per kilogram a day for a healthy body weight. Deficiency of protein can cause protein-energy malnutrition.

Energy balance and weight control—energy balance is energy intake minus energy output. Negative energy balance results in weight loss. Positive energy balance results in weight gain. A person with healthy weight shows good health. Obesity is total body fat percentages over 25 percent in men and 35 percent in women. A weight-loss program can be used to meet the dieter's nutritional needs. There are different kinds of treatments that can be used.

Nutrients, carbohydrates, lipids, and proteins can be calculated. It can also be referred from the food label or the cookbooks. The food label will have the detailed information, including daily value, carbohydrate, protein, lipid composition. It can be used to control weight and others according to the energy provided. Normal people can eat everything. Nutrition can make them healthily maintain weight control. It is important to patients. Nutrient imbalance can make them sick or even die. Dieting patients may limit their intake of carbohydrate, protein, and fats. People with heart disease will limit their intake of sodium from the food. Dieting people will need to calculate the calorie from the food to two thousand calories per day.

Diet

Diet is a food plan designed to maintain health and prevent and cure disease. It may follow the food guide pyramid and determine what amount of each nutrient is needed. It's easily understandable if you have a basic knowledge concerning their development and use. Food label is a good example of diet guide. The following must be listed: total kilocalories, kilocalories from fat, total fat, saturated fat, cholesterol, sodium, total carbohydrates, dietary fiber, sugars, protein, vitamin A, vitamin C, calcium, and iron. The information can then be used in diet planning.

The dietary guidelines emphasize changes that will reduce the risk of obesity, hypertension, cardiovascular disease, and diabetes. The dietary plan is not hard to implement and is not expensive. But the results may be disappointing even when you are following a diet change very closely. The reason may be due to management follow-up. Now, a management plan will be associated with the dietary plan so that the dietary plan will not be affected by mistakes such as a skipped meal.

A diabetic patient needs control of carbohydrates in food eating. A fixed amount of fifty grams to seventy grams of carbohydrates will be limited for each meal. Taking in more than the amount consumed will result in high or low blood sugar. It will affect the health of the patient. Food label reading will help the patient to control the carbohydrate taken. Family eating cannot be controlled by follow the diabetic recipe. Dining out is hard to control. Now, big fast food restaurants have nutrition information. In small restaurants, you need to do the control by yourself. You have to tell the waiter to use steaming or boiling instead of frying. Salad dressing needs to be put on the side of the plate. Portion control must be done. The time of food taking is important as late eating may affect blood sugar levels. Avoid busy hours of restaurant such that the time of eating can be estimated.

The common example is obesity.

1.   Look at the weight status.

        Measure the body mass index (BMI), weight/height square, and waist circumference. When the BMI is 25 or greater, health risk from obesity will begin.

2.   An action plan to change weight status.

        (I)   Become aware of the problem. By calculating the weight, we become aware of the problems. From here, we can find out more information about the cause of the problem and if we need to change exercise habits, levels of self-esteem, and a variety of other behaviors.

(a)   Look at the food diary; what are the factors influencing the eating habits? Do you eat due to stress, boredom, or depression? Eat too much or you dislike the wrong food?

(b)   From the eating pattern, can you decide on any change?

(II)   Set goal.

Set an achievable goal and allow a reasonable time to pursue it.

(III)   Measuring commitment.

Commitment is required in the success of behavioral change.

(IV)   Make a contract.

(V)   Psyching.

Psyching yourself up can enable you to progress toward your goals in spite of others' attitudes and opinions. No other person's words and actions can hurt you.

(VI)   Practicing the Plan.

The next step is to implement the plan. Monitor the plan. This can make you progress with the plan.

Try to avoid the problem/situation by controlling your food intake in events such as parties, coffee break.

(VII)   Reevaluating.

After practicing for a while, reassess the plan.

(VIII) Epilogue.

The overall success in the permanent change of habits, including quitting smoking, is motivation.

Usually, the weight loss plan will be best to reduce calories; moderating the amount of fat in the diet and engaging in regular physical activity are adequate for weight loss.

Fad Diet

Those diet plans cannot be carried out, and some can harm those who follow them. They are easily recognized, like quick weight loss. It cannot be permanent. It seems like fat loss. Actually, people lose mostly muscle and other lean tissue mass. As soon as they eat normally again, lost tissues are replaced, and the lost weight is back.

A diet plan mostly needs professional people like doctors and dietitians to help. The dietitian designs the plan for the different needs of people or patients. The doctor then monitors the patient's physical condition. Any deviation will be evaluated and corrected. The most important thing is to beware of a fad diet. It wastes time and may harm the body. In diabetes, for example, the diet plan can be controlled, but no fad plan can cure it.

Atmosphere and Service

Service

Food service has professional service training. They have orientation, a host, delivery food, computer, free food. Orientation will allow you to express what the company expects of them. It is better offered if there is a handbook that they can study the details of the company policy in. Hosting is a great way for your new employee to learn table numbers, take orders, and other table works. Delivery food is to know how to serve food. Computer is the most difficult work; you cannot rely on relationships to skip it. Know all the aspect of the functions of computer, then try phone calls and take to-go orders into the computer. Free food for the employees is the chance that the employees become familiar with the menu and the tastes of food. Later, they can recommend to the customers. The trainer has to make sure they can do everything before placing the staff on working, monitoring them before letting them do the job independently.

Atmosphere

You can feel the beautiful sensation when you enter the dining room. The pleasant atmosphere can cherish the ambience. This can make us enjoy a great dinner. The choice of food facilities are food, atmosphere and service, and price. For events like wedding, atmosphere is the most important consideration for choosing food service. Food becomes a helping role for the wedding event. The couple will be introduced to the guests. Their love story will be told and the guests bless them. Then, food will be served. The food can be very expensive or good food. Between the delivery of the courses of food, host will go to each table and thank the guests. The atmosphere is not mainly enjoy the food but to cerebrate the new wedding couples.

The factors of good atmosphere are location,music, lighting, décor, food service, customer, staff, and seating. These can creat good atmosphere to enjoy the food. Stress can affect people's appetite. Good location with easy parking, suitable music, beautiful lighting, ,décor can make you feel in a specific place,consumers are friendly, server are professional, and the seating is spacious, all can make the dining place like a wonderful area.

Locations—An easy find place can attract more people. Parking should be always available. A high class restaurant should be in a quiet area.

Music—It depends on the kind of customers and type of restaurant. if atmosphere is important, light music can be romantic for young people. Great music will be for events. No music needs for regular dinning.

Lighting—The light should be bright enough that people will not fell. Regular restaurant should be very bright. Restaurant with dancing can be darker.

Décor—It depends on what kind of environment you want to creat. Christmas should have Christmas tree and Christmas decoration.

Customers—should be well behaved and friendly. The next table noisy and swearing can affect your enjoyment of food and talking. All the time may be spent to stop them.

Server—must be professional. Friendly staff can attract more customers. They can take your order without mistakes. They can recommend you good food without cheat you order expensive food. They know how to serve you that food are in a good order and good temperatures.

Seating—should be spacious. People will not close with each other. The numbers of customers will bedefined in one table. A place will be saved for the servers to serve the table.

For religious people, they may have restrictions like vegetarian will not eat meats. They will pray before eat. This make sure the food is clean, the ambient is holy, the eating will follow the rule like no talking when eating. The result is psychological fit, physiological functions well, and the soul is holy.

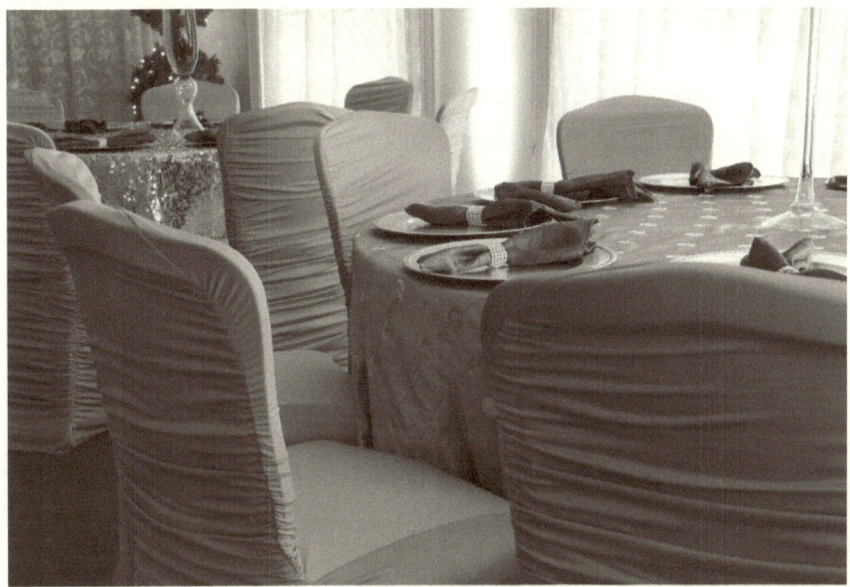

A family will not have service training. They learn it from the family or from experience. Hunger is the sensation of energy. Without food for a long time, muscle and fat will be broken down for energy by catabolysis. That's why starvation will make people thin. They will feel fatigued and dehydrated. Give them little water and then feed them food gradually. They will recover.

Mood can also affect appetite. People with bad moods don't want to eat. Those who are in a great mood will eat too much. Comfort food, like chocolate, may be provided. Religious people adopt a ceremony to maintain their mood. It's the spiritual food. Pray before you eat. It's great food desire, great digestion, and great spirit. When you go on an outdoor picnic or lunch, the air is fresh, the mountain is green, there is a blue sky, you can hear the flow of the river; it sets a great mood for lunch. Some people will enjoy an outdoor, spiritual, religious lunch.

Buddhist Meal

Buddhists mainly eat vegetables. Meat and fish are not allowed. Ten kinds of meats are avoided: humans, elephants, horses, dogs, snakes, lions, tigers, boars, and hyenas. Usually, at temples, chanting will be sung. When people feel a sense of hunger and peace, dinner will begin.

Zen Monk's Diet

In ancient China, the monks ate only two meals, one early and another around lunchtime. At evening, other monks will place a warm rock on their stomach to relieve the cold and hunger. Later, it evolves into an actual meal. Nowadays, the meal is more nourishing and palatable. The calorie comes from rice, the protein from tofu, and green tea is the beverage. In the morning, the monks have leftover rice, seasoned with soy sauce, served with plums and salt. A small cup of miso soup and a side dish of green vegetables are ready for the lunch. Evening meal is more luxurious, with fresh rice, pickles of choice, and two dishes. Miso soup will have tofu added. Cook the food by boiling, roasting, frying, and steaming, and eat the food fresh.

The ritual is based on nature. A chant is recited before the meal, which is eaten silently. Eating is done slowly; the monk concentrates on every taste and texture. Serve the food in five tastes by colorful presentation. Hot, sweet, bitter, salty, and sour match with five colors of yellow, white, black, red, and green. No food is left on the bowl; the last pickle is used to wipe the bowl clean.

Muslim Meal

They have definite guidelines on what can be eaten and what cannot be eaten. Prohibited food includes pork, any drink with alcohol in it, any human part, and birds of prey.

They have to follow a list of Muslim dietary practices.

- Recite the name of God, Allah, before eating and thank God after finishing.
- It is a good thing to eat by the right hand and in company.
- Think and contemplate in every item of food you eat by remembering God, the Creator, the Designer, the Organizer, and the Provider.
- It is important to eat when you are hungry.
- Don't eat in excess.
- Halal foods are recommended.

Vegetables are not restricted. Fasting is considered an opportunity to wipe off the sins. It's a chance to understand the hunger of poor people. It can also control appetite and help avoid food addiction. Fasting lasts from dawn to sunset, as all food and drink are absent.

Christian Dining

Most Christians are omnivores and have no restrictions in meat. Sometimes they will fast for religious reasons. Table decorations will include violets, candles, and angel figurines. Violet is a symbol of humility. Candles can be treated as prayer candles. They are of different size and colors. Angels are Christian symbols.

Christmas parties can be held on the Christmas holiday. There are no strict sets of rules. Turkey is the most popular food. It will be surrounded by mashed potatoes, gravy, bread rolls, cranberry sauce, pumpkin pie, spiral-cut ham, and roasted beef. Add corn bread, green beans, mixed salad, fried tofu, and cheese. Onion soup or tomato soup will be a good idea. Dessert includes coleslaw, red velvet cake.

The Christians will begin worship when the food is ready and put on the tables. Someone will lead the prayer, usually the pastor. They thank God for the food. Then, they begin to enjoy the food and cheer. Usually, the food is prepared by catering.

The spiritual food not only gives you physical satisfaction of hunger, but also works as a spiritual mood activator. It can make you more healthy.

Price

Since markets vary considerably, a buyer must know the characteristics of the local market. This requires the investigation of market supplies of all types. The kinds of products, costs, supply and demand, and services provided must be studied. Then, the buyer must determine the amount and kind of food to be purchased. Today, it is quicker and easier to use the Internet to place the order and the telephone to do the negotiation. After delivery, stocks are kept up to a desired level. The expiration must be checked to ensure they will be used up before the last day. Any food after the expiration day should be discarded.

Standard of quality is important. Standards have been established for many foods by the US Department of Agriculture (USDA). They indicate the various characteristics of a specific grade of items. Three or more grades may be used, and in each the quality characteristic will be different. So the buyer can assess the quality of the food without having to examine it. Meat, poultry, eggs, butter, and fresh or processed fruits and vegetables are often graded. A fresh product needs visual inspection. Fish should smell good, and the eyes are clear. Meat should not smell bad if put on the tables too long.

Food facilities need to calculate the different costs, like the labor and food costs. They may simply add the profit to the cost in deciding the price. Then, they must evaluate the purchase. Families can have a shopping list. A supermarket coupon book is a must-have. Discounted products will be purchased first. A budget for every meal will be estimated first. All purchases will be limited to the budget. Extra purchases will be restricted. The budget must be followed tightly. The purchase may be daily, weekly, or monthly due to the usage and expiration date of food.

After the purchase, food should be stored according to their meal planning. The other storage is based on their characteristic. Meat, fish, poultry, egg, vegetables, and milk should be stored in a refrigerator. Frozen foods should be stored in a freezer. The space of the refrigerator depends on the food and meals served. It needs to be cleaned often. Air circulation can make the refrigerator work properly. The temperature in different parts of a refrigerated area may vary. Perishable foods should be stored in the coldest area, which is *near the bottom*. The temperature should be checked frequently using the thermometer.

If you are eating outside, the price and rating of the restaurant should be checked first. Personal referral will be the best. The price appears to be lower than the cost of making your own food at home. Only on important days like birthdays or festivals will expensive restaurants be chosen.

Food is a fixed cost of life. If the expense cannot be kept, the financial situation of the family will be worse. A good budget should be formulated with the meal planning. Then, the budget needs to be carried out accurately.

The Four Factors of the Quality of Food

The high quality of food is the combination of characteristics in a product that makes it acceptable to a large number of people. These may include price, convenience, location, service, sensory, healthfulness of food, social or physical environment or atmosphere, and sanitation. Thus, people like McDonald's, Burger King, KFC, and Pizza Hut. That is, people like hamburger, pizza, chicken because of their convenience, fast service, and low price. Actually, the quality of food will be considered first. Second is the service. Last is the price.

The high quality of food is determined by four factors. They are marketing, social, psychological, and chemical-physical aspects. These factors must be integrated to produce satisfying products.

Marketing—as the number of food service restaurant grows fast, more people will eat outside. Food service offers fixed numbers of food. This can offer the availability of food at a controlled cost; also, demographic data indicates that the food service is meeting the needs of some market segments better than others are. There are different kinds of competition. Famous food service will promote known brands of foods. Family-dining restaurants will promote catering to children. However, most of the people will still dine at home. They are lower in price, convenient, and free to cook and eat without formal etiquette.

Social influence—it's the social trends and lifestyles. Consumers' mobility and their contacts with diverse cultures expand their exposure to different foods. Social trends develop global culture and lifestyle. Recent trends are increasing interest in casual dining at table service restaurants, interest in ethnic or national foods with Italian, Chinese, or Mexican. People are also concerned with nutrition and health. The trend to eat away from home cannot replace family dining at home The differences in various situations are in the amount of time allocated to eating, the amount of relaxation and entertainment associated, and the cost.

Psychological influences—the quality of food is a personal perception based on interrelated psychological, physiological, environmental, and emotional factors associated with one's heritage and family. For these reasons, the mother's cooking may not be the same without home and the mother; even the mother's recipe is followed precisely. Food is the same, but the atmosphere of eating is different. The taste and smell are different. There is something special that can only be found in the food. The perception of food quality associated with food memories is important in their life. The positive psychological association is necessary to make the quality high.

Physical-chemical influence—sensory characteristics of food are a part of overall quality perception. We perceive these characteristics by our senses of taste, touch, sight, smell, and hearing. Those senses of color, clarity, gloss, and appearance are related to sight; (2) flavor is related to taste; and (3) texture is related to mouth feel.

Color—we perceive color with our eyes, and light and the chemical and physical properties of food affect the perception. A human eye has the ability to see within only a particular area of wavelength on the electromagnetic spectrum, called the visible region. Light has the color that is dependent upon the composition of the wavelength, and this will affect the color we see. Particular colors can be derived from different wavelengths and by mixing lights. Food evaluation should always be done with lighting similar to daylight. The chemical and physical properties of food are important to color perception. Properties that influence color are pigments and the density of the material. Pigments that impart color include chlorophylls (green), anthocyanins (blue red), and heme (red brown). Pigments in conjunction with food density affect the behavior of light and an observer's view of color and appearance. Since our eyes are a principle factor in perceiving color, the value of analysis with instruments are limited, and food color evaluation for product development may better be done by consumers of food.

Flavor—food flavor is a function of chemical composition, physiological perception, psychological perception, and training. Chemicals affect flavor at the levels of elements, compound, gross substance, and the synergy of substance, The element, Na, sodium; S, sulfur; C, carbon; and Cl, chlorine, for example, have profound effects on taste. Chemical compound gives flavor to food. For example, xanthines give bitter flavor in caffeine and tannin. Physiologically, taste is perceived through the papillae on the tongue. Sweet, sour, bitter are the basic tastes that people are able to perceive. However, this can be sensed in innumerable combinations and degrees of intensity to greatly enhance taste perception. In addition, saliva makes a contribution to taste by dissolving and releasing the flavors of food constituents. Aroma is another physiologic factor of taste. Some of what the brain integrates to perceive as taste is based on our olfactory sense in the nose. The external aroma of roasted meat is indistinguishable from the contribution of aroma perceived in the mouth while eating. Training in tasting is important in individual taste perception. This can be trained to identify precise flavors, intensity of particular flavor components, and the time of flavor perception. The time of flavor perception is important in aftertaste and in the manufacture of items such as chewing gum where sucking or chewing releases flavor over time. Analysis of food is highly important to quality control and product development and is a skill that can be learned through experience and careful thought.

Texture—it's the structure and organization of food. Texture can be perceived through the eyes and through the sense of touch, particularly in the mouth. Structural characteristics include hardness, smoothness, toughness, and consistency. The texture of food is directly related to distinguishing characteristics and acceptability. Thus, foods hard to break apart as meat are tough. Texture is extremely important in food acceptability. In food development and quality control, these must be selected in an individual basis.

Other senses—sound, spiciness, and temperature are other factors related to the sense and acceptance. The sound of crispness when food is eaten probably makes a big contribution. Snack foods that do not crunch or make other noises when consumed probably are not crispy and, thus, lack acceptability. Depending on an individual's own senses of taste and touch, food may be spicy or hot in temperature to the point of being physically irritating and painful to eat. Acceptable spiciness and temperature are purely personal. While some people prefer very hot spices and very hot temperature, others find these characteristics irritating.

These factors of food quality determine our love of food. And your mother knows your preference very well and makes the great food for you. Thus, many people will remember the food that is made by their mother and love it. It can last for a long time.

Food service will make the food lower in price and served fast and modified to fit the culture, climate, and appetite of the group of people they serve. Individual tastes cannot be considered, like diet-food people (e.g., diabetic people). So daily family and regional meals cannot be replaced.

When friends or religious people have a gathering, they will love the same food. After praying, the soul enters the mind. You will recall the deliciousness of the food you enjoyed before. When eating, it will be the same as you expect. Digestion is great. It can make you more energetic.

Hunger can create desire for food. Starvation can make people thin as muscles are broken down into energy. The appetite will not be considered as we will not choose food. Quality of food is not important.

Most of the time, we will be affected by these four factors of the quality of food. They determine our eating life. They subconsciously or consciously influence our eating patterns and habits.

The Best Food

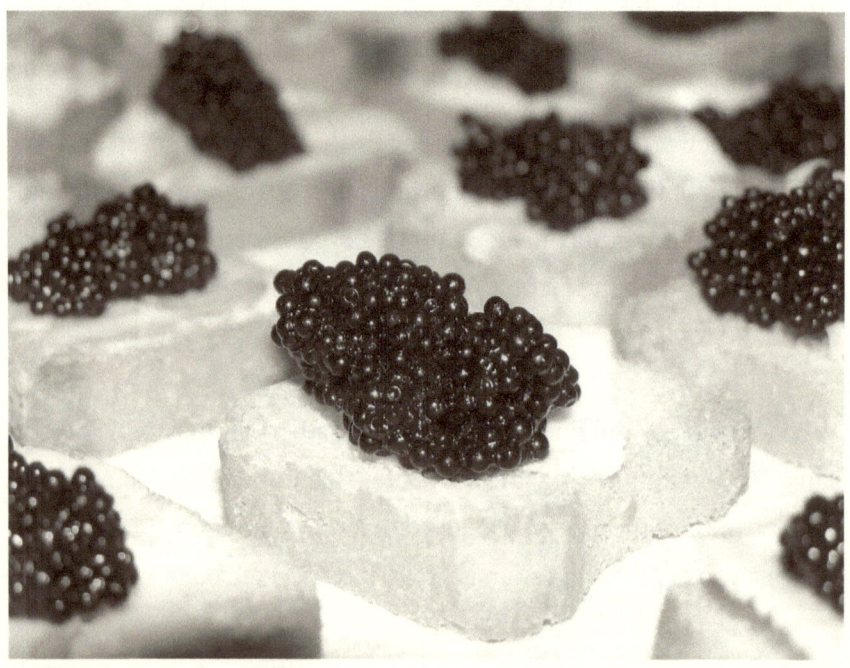

It may be delicious, rare, good for health, expensive, and or for medical use. It can be birds, animals, fish, insect, or even microorganisms. Thus, donkey is a delicious animal. A shark's fin is expensive. Wild vegetable was a rare food during wartime. Raw fish, raw meat are not sanitary but now are the best restaurant food after special handling.

We need food for providing energy for us to perform activities. Without food, with no more energy, we will feel hungry. Our body will break down the muscle to supply energy. That's why hungry people will be thin. We need about two thousand calories per day. When we are hungry, we can eat anything. When our livings are better, we need appetite. It will not only satisfy our hunger, but will also make it enjoyable. It will provide our physical need for energy. The color of food matches the aromatic smell in frying the food and the taste of the food. After praying, the atmosphere is peaceful or entertaining for people to enjoy the food. With the wonderful surrounding, the light is tender, the spacious area makes it feel comfortable, music is light such that can comfort the mind. It is like being on a green countryside with the courtyard paintings on the walls. The mind, the body, and the soul coincide with it. Eating is a perfect enjoyment.

Food can also function to strengthen our body, to prevent and cure disease. It's the nutrition and diet of food. A well-balanced meal of different kinds of meat, vegetables, grains, and poultry is enough for our daily use. Diet is for a sick patient. It needs to be calculated in the kind and amount of food prepared and consumed.

Supplements of food can strengthen our body. A vitamin is one of the supplements. There are vitamins A, B, C, D, E, K, and so on. They can regulate our body functions. It can come from food or pills. Popular carrot juice can provide vitamin A. Vegetable juice can provide vitamin C. A mineral is another kind of supplement. It can also come from pills or food. Generally, it can strengthen our body.

Food can cause disease and prevent diseases. Aloe can prevent cancer. The juice is stored in the refrigerator, and you drink it every day. It is not toxic, so it will not have side effects. It is safe to drink. Some food combinations can cause disease. Lamb mixed with watermelon will affect breathing. Onion and honey together will hurt the eyes. Rabbit and vegetable, pak choy, will cause vomiting. Potatoes and banana will hurt the skin. Soya bean and egg will cause constipation. Tofu and honey will hurt one's hearing. Tomato and cucumber will hurt the stomach. Before, it is by experience; now, it can be tested by chemical analysis.

Food can heal diseases. Fiber can prevent and cure intestine cancer. Oysters can lower blood pressure. Tea can prevent stomachache. Coffee can prevent breathing problems. Milk is rich in calcium. Drinking it every day is good for the bones. Traditional doctors will add herbs to the food to cure disease. Ginger added to Coca-Cola can heal coughing. Diet is a planned food program that can heal disease. Salt over a certain amount can cause high blood pressure. Food containing high amounts of carbohydrates can raise sugar levels. Food carbohydrates need to be consumed under a certain amount for every meal to be healthy. There are no formulas for diet food in order for one to keep fit. Some eat green apples everyday to keep fit. That may or may not work. Eating vegetables or fiber is healthy and will keep you fit.

Some foods are expensive. Some foods are cheap but high in nutritional value. The following are very interesting high-cost foods and high-nutritional-value foods.

Matsutake mushrooms are expensive, about $1,000/pound because of their rarity. They grow in Japan.

Densuke watermelons grow on the northern island of Hokkaido in Japan and cost $6,100, also because of their rarity. They are a type of black watermelons about seventeen pounds heavy. They are used as a gift. They are harder and crisper and have a different level of sweetness.

Almas caviar comes from Iran; its rarity and expensiveness make it cost $25,000. It sells a kilo in a 24K gold in London, England's Piccadilly named Caviar House & Prunier. Thus, the meal is the most expensive in Britain. They also sell an affordable small-size tin for $1,250.

Italian white alba truffles are notoriously pricey because they are hard to cultivate. They are called king of all fungi. A gigantic Italian white alba truffle was sold for $160,406.

The other expensive general foods are more affordable due to the fact that supply will be plenty. Thus, a thousand-year old ginseng will cost $10,000. A taste tea per ounce may cost $10,000. A rare and big rod fish or a snake may cost several hundred dollars.

Ginger is cheap, but it has high medicinal value.

Tofu is high in protein.

Tea is tasteful. It can be used for enjoyment of life. Like English afternoon tea, it is served in social gatherings. Religious people use it for meditation.

Besides natural food, there are also artificial foods. They can be food additives like food coloring. Food can also be preserved like canning, freezing, thermal processing, moisture control, ionizing radiation. After preserving, the food can be stored for a longer time. There are also organic foods. Those are mainly vegetables grown without pesticides. There are also gene foods that can supply the need of the growth of population of people.

Cooking

There are plenty of natural and artificial foods to choose. With the advancement of science, different foods in different areas can be transported to different places in a short time. With a meal plan of three meals every day, a menu and shop list of food are planned.

Food can be prepared in advance or at mealtime. It depends on the tools available. The methods may be frying, steaming, simmering, or boiling. Without liquid, it can be baking, grilling, roasting, and broiling. Pastries like bread and cake will use baking. The meals may include pantry items, stocks, soups, and sauces. The materials can be meat, poultry, fish, and vegetables. It can be raw consumption or cooking for safety reasons. Drinks may be soda, milk, beer, and wine.

Before you prepare the food, a recipe is important. Some housewives don't have a recipe. It is all by experience. They can also ask people. If they still don't know how to prepare food, maybe they can ask people to show them or guide them or coach them to cook the food. They learn one by one, like mothers and daughters do. After practice, they can cook the food that the family will like. Some will follow a recipe. But usually the recipe is not detailed. Many important points will be omitted.

We can write or rewrite a recipe. It is formula, standardized for the quality of the food.

Writing a Recipe

1. Select an item—record exact quantities of ingredients, procedures, equipment, portion sizes, yield, and specifications.

2. Test for quality and yield.

3. Adjust in terms of usual quantities to be prepared, portion size, yield, institutional weights or measures, institutional purchase units, and quality.

4. Prepare in terms of adjustment.

5. Prepare, adjust, and evaluate as many times as necessary to achieve the quality and cost standard desired.

It then can be tested until it is satisfactory. If they have interest, they can find out more. They have friends retiring from restaurant service. They can form an informal apprentice relationship to learn the standard restaurant food. One-on-one training can ensure the result is good. Make sure you can reproduce the food exactly. Company cooking training can also train you as a good cook required by the food facilities. You need to produce the food as required by the restaurant. Usually, they will differentiate the jobs such that some are trained as pantry cooks, others are sauté cooks, frying cooks, etc. Cooking school can make you learn more of the principles of cooking so that you can cook everything. But it depends on the cooking school. Some just let you do the cooking by following the recipe. Some cooking schools have hands-on training. You can learn by following them cook the same food to make sure they are the same. Cooking school also requires you to study the theory and principles of cooking. Further development of the students to work as cooks or cooking instructors or to open a restaurant depends on the school. They have the human resource department to help students.

With the menu, the recipe, the shop list of purchase, your meal planning is done. You can cook for and serve the family.

Service can be seated or buffet service. There are seated American, English, or French-style services. Usually, it's mixed style or freestyle. In the American style, it is the women who sit first, then elderly men, children, and finally, men. Breads and butter are on the table. During the meal, people can begin to talk.

One must know how to eat good food. Pairing wine and food can make the food more enjoyable. Usually, red wine is for meat, white wine for fish. Caviar can be spooned for eating. A soup can use 85 percent of a spoon's surface in order for one to enjoy it. A salad can use a fork to roll it. Meat can be cut into small pieces for eating. Fish can be cut into pieces, and a fork can be used to hold it. The meat from lobsters and oysters can be separated from the shell first; next, it can be cut for you to eat. Without you knowing how to eat, eating cannot be fully enjoyed. You can ask people how to eat. Generally, the food service facilities can tell you how to eat. The etiquette will be omitted as people prefer to use any way they like to eat, even use the hand. Of course, sometimes, using the proper way of eating can make you enjoy the food and is good for your health. Eating too fast may hurt your digestive system. Eating under stress, like eating with your disliked boss, may harm your health and appetite.

Meal Planning

(a)   Menu Planning

It includes budget, food purchase, how many people, how many courses.

Usually, it will be breakfast, lunch, dinner, and snack time. What will be in the breakfast? It may be simply as bread and butter. The more luxurious will include egg, ham, and potato. Coffee and tea will be served.

Lunch will be a little more but fast-food-style. It may be a soup; salad; main dish of fish; beef, or pork; and finally, a dessert and coffee.

Dinner will be the big one as people have more time to enjoy. It may be buffet-style or an individual choice. A soup is a good starting point. A basket of bread and salad will be good appetizers. Next, choose fish, meat, and poultry. Wine will accompany the selection all the way. Coffee, tea, and soda will be served as refreshments. Finally, it's the dessert of ice cream and fruits of bananas, apples, and oranges.

Nutrition must be balanced. The food guide can be used. The bottom level is fruits, the middle one is for the meat, fish, and the top one is for fatty food. The cost will be limited to less than $100/day.

It begins with a meal planner. On weekdays, it should be breakfast and dinner. Usually, people eat lunch outside. The housewife can add lunch. Dining out should be allowed any time to substitute any meal. The number of meals depends on breakfast, lunch, or dinner and the number of people. Breakfast can be very casual, with milk or juice ready and with bread and butter on the table. Lunch will be fewer courses, including soup, salad, main dish, and coffee. Dinner will have more courses, including a starter, soup, main dish, salad, dessert, and refreshments of coffee or wine. It can be eaten together or left for late workers to enjoy by heating it up.

A shop list for the supermarket should be prepared. Flyers of supermarket will be checked to find out the cheapest price of food. It can be canned, frozen, or fresh. Leftovers can be used again to prepare the food. Usually, a week of food is enough, and make sure it will not be stored longer than its used date.

A menu will make the meal planning more practical and left with more choices. It includes three meals a day for a week or a month. It can be cyclic. For festivals, you can add a big meal, like for Thanksgiving.

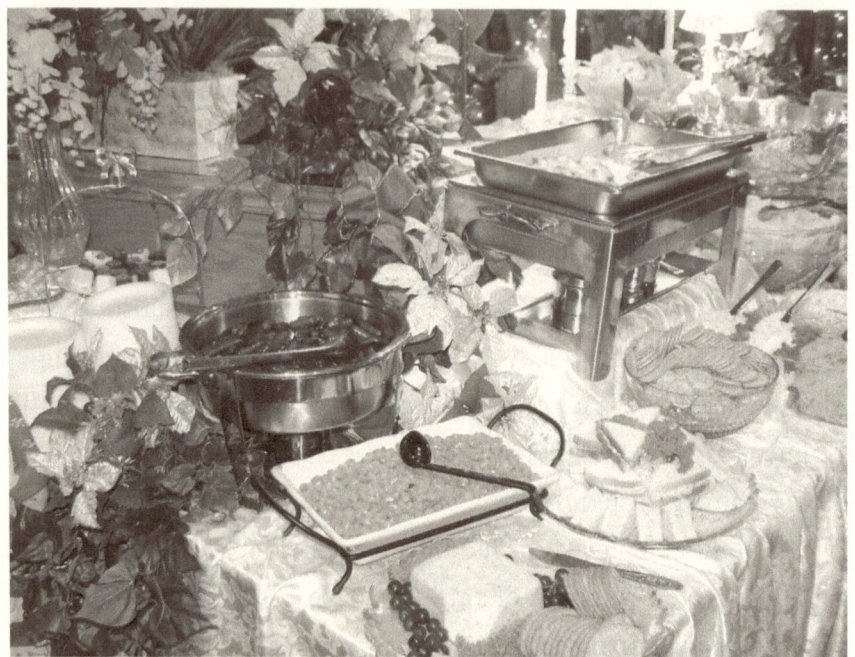

Menu planning can save time and money and is nutritious. It reduces trips to the supermarket, reduces impulse spending. You can buy bulk produce. No need to go back to the supermarket for missing items. Balanced nutrition can be planned. It is better than planning close to meal time. If you plan too later, you may be find missing ingredients for a course of meal.

Traditional American Dinner for Six

Corn and clam chowder

Peppercorn steaks with sauce

Baked potatoes with gravy

Steamed vegetable

Fried salmon fish fillet

Angel food cake with fresh mango

The chowder soup calls for frozen, canned, or fresh corn. The steaks are served with potatoes and steamed broccoli. Angel food cake can be purchased for convenience. They are served with a sliced mango. The menu can then be checked by the members of the household. It can be modified.

Sometimes, a festival meal can be prepared in the menu, like Thanksgiving, with turkey as the main dish.

Thanksgiving

Oven-roasted turkey with a stuffing of bread, sage, chopped celery, onions

Mashed potatoes

Macaroni and cheese

Salad

Bread and pie

Pork and beans

Fruits

Coffee, tea, and wine

It's the feast between the Pilgrims and Native Indians. It includes turkey, waterfowl, fish, seafood, pumpkin, and squash. Now, modern Thanksgiving feast has been modified. A turkey takes a long time to cook, but you can buy one. Tea and coffee need to be ready after serving food. It is a religious feast where some rules must be followed.

This can be a sample of a menu. The courses can be added or subtracted. It is easier to follow as everything is well planned. The food materials are ready. Some are ready-made food. You just cook it and enjoy it.

(b)   Meal Planning

After we choose the kinds of food by their food quality, we will plan the meals. The food must be smelled good with aroma, be colorful matching, be delicious, be healthy, be sanitized for safety, and be served in good atmosphere without gaining negative feedback. The making of food is determined by how much the family have consumed. What is the amount of food and the kind of food we will buy? At what price will we buy? The quality of food purchased will be controlled by inspection. Food must meet specifications graded by the US Department of Agriculture. Other inspections of freshness will be done through personal knowledge and experience. How do you cook them and plan the time of cooking? Recipes can be followed from the cookbook or modified or made into new ones. It can standardize the consistent quality of food. How is it eaten? Should we eat together or eat buffet-style?

Three meals will be planned each day. Breakfast will be casual as people have no time to enjoy it. Lunch may be skipped as many people will eat outside. Only for dinner will people stay at home to eat. It should be a good one as people have time to enjoy the food. A snack depends on each person's habit. Family members can choose what food to eat. It can follow the meal plan designed by food professionals. It may be based on what is delicious or for health reasons.

Cooking can be done by remembering from experience or following a recipe. Recipes cannot be perfect and detailed. Sometimes, we follow them, but the product is still a mess. By our experience, we can rewrite it, but the product may be a different one.

Writing a Recipe

1. Select a dish—record the exact quantity of ingredients, procedures, equipment, portion size, yield, and specifications. Practically, just see what you have. Decide the size of food for the people present at dinner.
2. Test for quality and yield—we need to know the yield to meet needs of the number of people eating.
3. Adjust in terms of usual quantities to be prepared, portion sizes, yield, institutional weights or measures, institutional purchase units, and quality. Practically, you can estimate this.
4. Prepare in terms of adjustments. It can fit all the people by changing a little of the recipe.
5. Prepare, adjust, and evaluate as many times as necessary to achieve the quality and cost standard desired.

Some will follow a recipe. Luckily, the food will be the one they expect or, if not, a mess. Some will learn by one-on-one training, like mothers and daughters do. After practice, you can cook those foods that the family will like. Varieties of food can be more than you have served before.

Family eating is freestyle. It can be table-style or a buffet. It can be catered or a banquet. It can be informal. You can have a movie show or a magic show at the time of eating. You can also have karaoke after food enjoyment.

Food service facilities will use an operational concept. This includes the theme, decor, type of service, price structure, kind of menu items, entertainment, general atmosphere, and other unique features like spiritual, religious food. You have to pray before you can eat. Some have light music. After eating, you can talk or enjoy the atmosphere. Some have shows, live jazz music, or a magic show. The kind of operation determines what foods are developed, the organization of preparation procedures, and the basic food cost. Thus, steak, hamburger, and children's items will have distinct cost and quality characteristics related to service in fast food, family, or gourmet restaurants. It is important to note that food must meet the customer's expectations, which have been advertised by the food service. The opening is based on extensive market research and has occurred with a great deal of media flourish.

Family members can eat the way they like or follow the family practice. It can be easily as a person's meal or a family's meal. The family may be formal as guests are invited. It depends on the culture and habit of the guest. The etiquette may be the common one or rely on the culture of the people eating.

Breakfast, Lunch, Dinner, and Banquet

They are traditional events. Except for banquet, there's no reason you have to follow etiquette rules. Food can be American food, ethnic food, vegetarian food, or famous food, like melting pot. Many people want to try the fondue. Of course, they will later try the Chinese hot pot. It's for a different appetite.

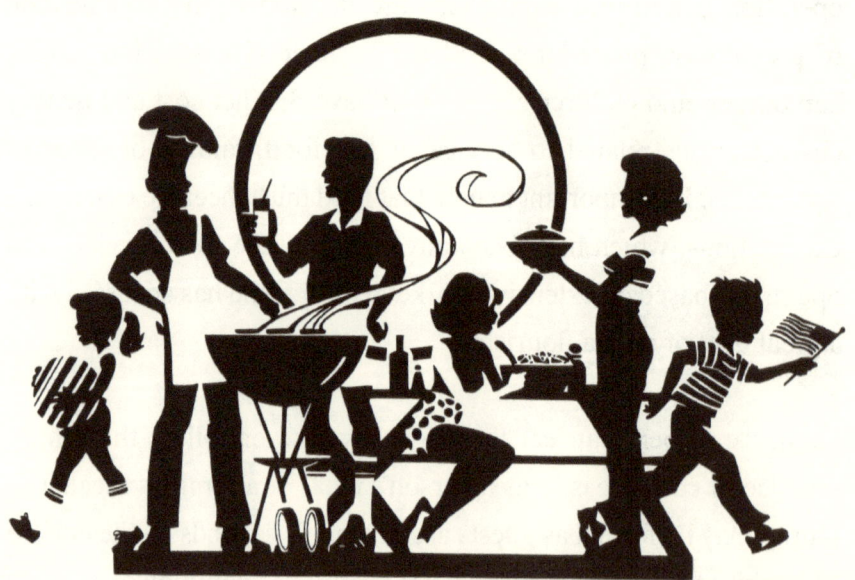

Usually, the breakfast is a three-course meal. Lunch and dinner are six-course meals. The food may be paired with wines. The breakfast usually will be served with orange juice or milk. Then comes the scrambled egg or pancake or ham. At last, it's the coffee.

The lunch is eaten fast as many people have limited time. Fast food is the first choice. Some restaurants provide a special lunch menu. A luxury restaurant has à la carte or California menu, which can be called an all-purpose menu fitting three meals. Usually, it's a three- to four-course meal. The first is salad or soup or cocktail or red or white wine. The second one is a main entrée of choice of steak, pizza, hamburger, beef, pork chop, or chicken. The last one is dessert and coffee.

Dinner is the most formal one because people have plenty of time. Exclusive restaurants for people, one or two, will provide light music, candlelight. Family dinner will have jazz band music. Birthday cakes or discounts will be offered for senior people or birthday celebrators. They may need to check the identification. The best partnership in history was that of Escoffier and Ritz. Escoffier managed the kitchen while Ritz took care of the front. Escoffier was a great chef and the executive chef. He developed food ideas and preparation. He perfected the organization of workers in the kitchen. He wrote a great cookbook that is used today. *Ritzy* means "elegant, ostentatious, fancy, or fashionable." The informal leaders of culture, society, politics, the arts, and science became patrons of these two men.

First, hosts invite guests into their living room and serve them light alcoholic drinks and small appetizers to stimulate their appetites for the meal ahead. The serving of aperitif is also a warm and friendly gesture, indicating the hosts' pleasure at having guests over for dinner. Waiting for latecomers becomes more bearable in this relaxed environment. A glass of champagne or cocktail will be served at arrival or during the first course. A basket of bread, nuts, and crackers is served alongside these alcoholic beverages. Then soup will be served, like French onion soup. The third course is meat or fish with a side dish of salad, rice, or pasta. Wine is served throughout the meal. Red wine is for red meat, while white wine is for white meat or fish. The fourth is the chess board of varying textures and flavors. Then, dessert will be served, like chocolate mousse. The last one is coffee. Coffee is served in a relaxed atmosphere of the living room. Each customer is served coffee in a small cup, accompanied by a square piece of dark chocolate, which can enhance the aroma and taste of coffee. At the end of the dinner, guests are offered a small drink of strong alcoholic beverages such as cognac, brandy, or whisky. In festivals like the ones with Christmas dinner, guests will be offered cigars to puff on.

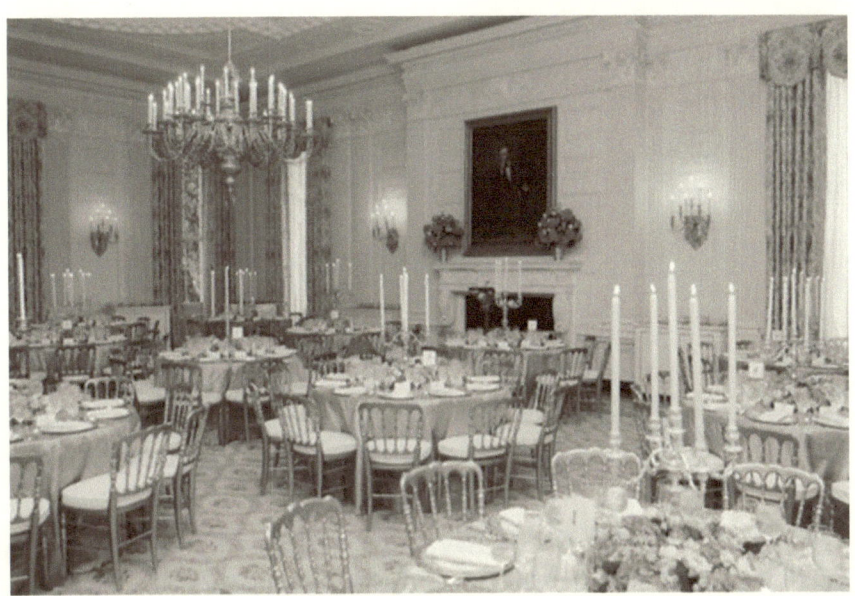

A typical White House dinner menu for review, its simple elegance reflects Escoffier's influence.

Courtesy of chefs Haller and Bender of the White House.

Dinner

Johannisberger Klaus

1970   Timbale of Seafood White House
Fleurons Dore'es

Louis Martini   Cha'teaubriand Be'arnaise
Caberenet Sauvignon   Pommes Souffle'es
1968   Artichokes Andalouse

Bible Lettuce salad
Brie Chess
Dom Pe'rignon   French Peaches Glace'es Manticello
1964   sauce Framboise

The White house
Tuesday, July 24, 1973.

Ethnic Dinner

They spent a lot of money on decoration, sea view, mountain view, small yard view, luxury wallpaper, crystal light, luxury silver utensils. It's the enjoyment of life, not food only. You can see from outside of the culture they promote. The server may wear traditional clothes. The eating will still be American style (i.e., using a fork, a spoon, and a knife, instead of using the hand or other tools). A popular one will be the hot pot. The restaurant provides a hot pot with soup base. They also provide meat, seafood, vegetables. You can then put them piece by piece into the boiling soup to cook. It's a pleasure to cook by yourself to the point that you like to practice and try.

Street Dinner or Snack

The food cart will provide a lot of choices of simple food, like sandwich, hot dog, fruit salad, chips, a drink of soda, and coffee. They are fast or ready food. You don't have to wait.

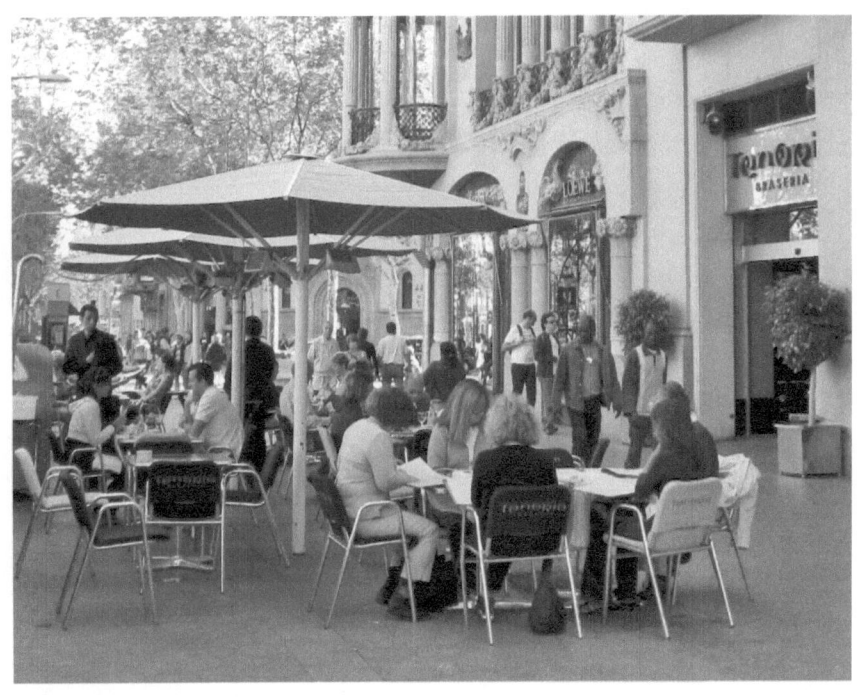

Convenience Food

Those are found in a convenience store. They may be ready-made or semi-ready food. You can use the microwave oven to cook the food. There are more choices of food. There are different kinds of drinks, but you cannot drink alcoholic drinks like beer or wine there.

Fast Food

Usually, in formal dinners, one will not choose fast food.

Religious Food

Some have strict rules to follow, like Muslims and Buddhists. The food is limited, the drink is limited, and the etiquette is formal. Before they eat, they pray or chant to make the dinner more spiritual. Some have a witch dance and sing to pray for love, wealth, and health.

The Best Breakfast

Chambord has the best breakfast, which costs $35,000. It begins with a hand-decorated, bejewelled croissant covered in edible gold and diamonds and is followed by hand-seeded jam and a cup of *kopi luwak*. The last one is champagne cocktail. The costs mainly rely on the decorations.

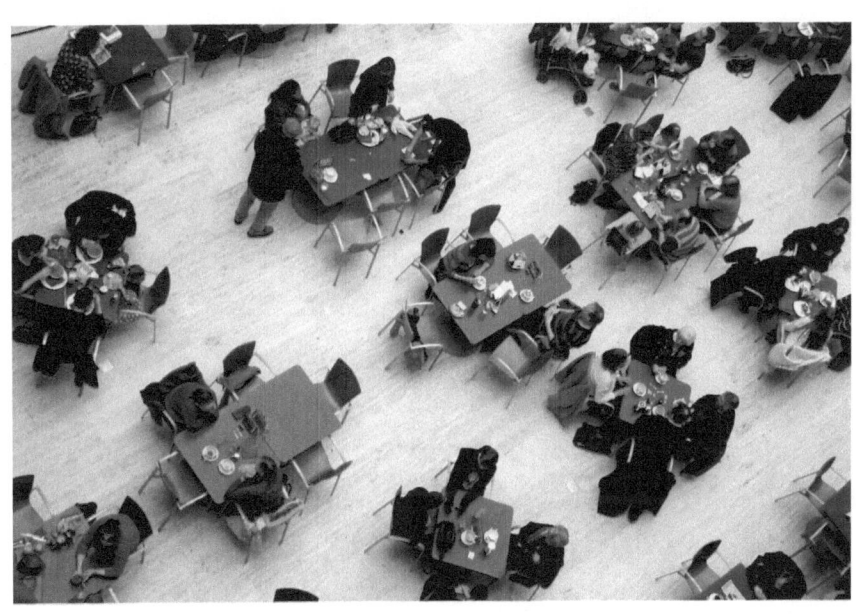

The Best Lunch

It is from Château Mouton Rothschild, patron of the world's most expensive lunch with the company of billionaire investor and philanthropist Warren Buffett. It includes an entrée laden with gold flake and white truffle, foie gras, or a cabernet sauvignon. This power lunch was hosted to benefit Glide Foundation, a charity organization. It records over $2.5 million in profit.

The Best Dinner

A Christmas dinner for four cooked by British chef Ben can cost $200,000. The meal begins with a bottle of Diva Vodka and a bottle of Piper Heidsieck 1907 champagne. Each course is paired with a wine. The first one is a bird's nest full of Almas caviar with 150-year-old balsamic vinegar and *jamón pata negra ibérico*. The second is a whole white alba truffle served with a melon from China. The meal's centerpiece is a rare breed of turkey served with Wagyu beef heart and fillet served with Périgord truffles and pistachios. And it is all wrapped in a gold leaf. Dessert is served on a gold Ugandan vanilla plate and incorporates the beans of coffee berries and Densuke watermelons from Japan.

The Best Catering

The most common event that requires catering is the wedding. The most elegant and formal catering service is plated service. This is the catering service that prepares the food and serves the guest at the table side. The cost includes preparation, delivering, serving, bus the table, and clean all the dishes. It is like your one-time own restaurant. All the work is done for you. You are free to enjoy the event, and everything is taken care of without you having to worry about any details while you are busy with the event. The one for President Clinton cost $750,000.

The other one is buffet service. Guests set up and stand in a line and serve for themselves. It's a less-expensive way. Food is prepared and arranged on a buffet table where your guests can help themselves to what they like. Depending on the type and quantity of food, you may prefer to have your staff serve on the buffet line. This helps to ensure that service plates and trays are refilled promptly and the buffet tables are kept looking attractive. The economic one is to-go. You pick up, deliver, set up, and service. Later, clean up and return any service items after the event. This is appropriate for those events when you can't know in advance exactly what time your people may be ready to eat.

No matter what kind of meal, it must have something that can attract you. It may be rare food, dining with president or for charity, gold and decoration with jewelry. Usually, it only lasts one time. First, it is expensive. Second, it takes a lot of time.

Banquet

Banquet is fun. It can be for a wedding and event, a birthday, a funeral, or any special celebration. The most important one is the wedding. Some hotels have wedding packages including pickup, the wedding cake, a banquet, and the honeymoon room.

Banquet can be like catering. All the foods are placed on the table. Then, there is singing and dancing. Guests can chat around with their friends. It can be a formal banquet serviced by the food-service provider. The host addresses the guest about the new couple, how they met and finally married. Then, food is served one by one. It can be American food like salad, main entrée, and dessert. Coffee and wine are served at a reception table. It can be ethnic food, depending on the culture of the parties. Finally, a farewell reception will be held to thank the guests. The atmosphere will be entertaining, and the host's brother and sister will try to play and have fun with the new couples.

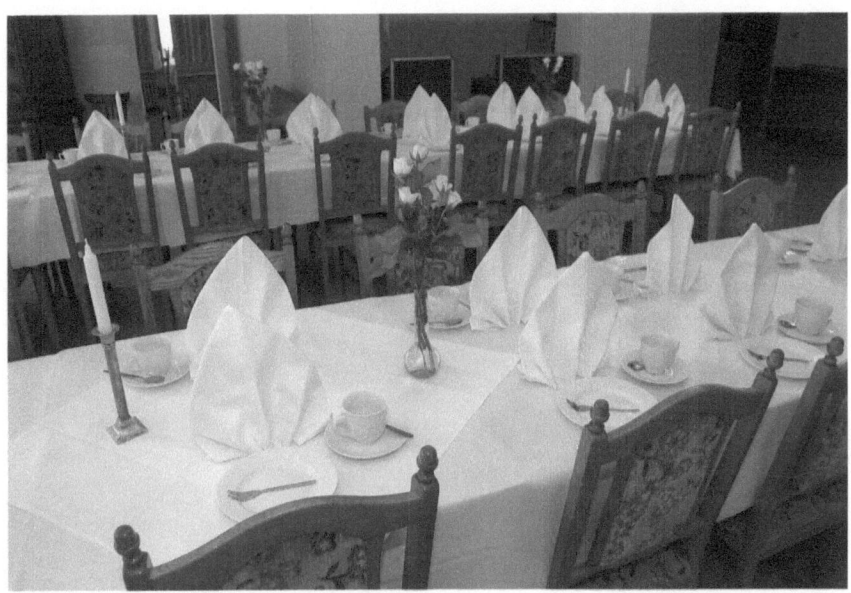

A banquet was held for the senior people before. It was thousands of table of banquet. The host first addressed the guest and wished them long life. Singers were invited to sing the birthday song. There were variety shows, like a cardinal party. The atmosphere was impressive. Many people went in and out. Temporary restrooms were stationed at the roadside. People speaking to one another sometimes had to shout. It was fun. The food was traditional food, a big bowl of a mixture of different kinds of food. It included meat, seafood, vegetables, and many dried seafood. The climax was the raffle. Almost everyone got a prize.

French Banquet

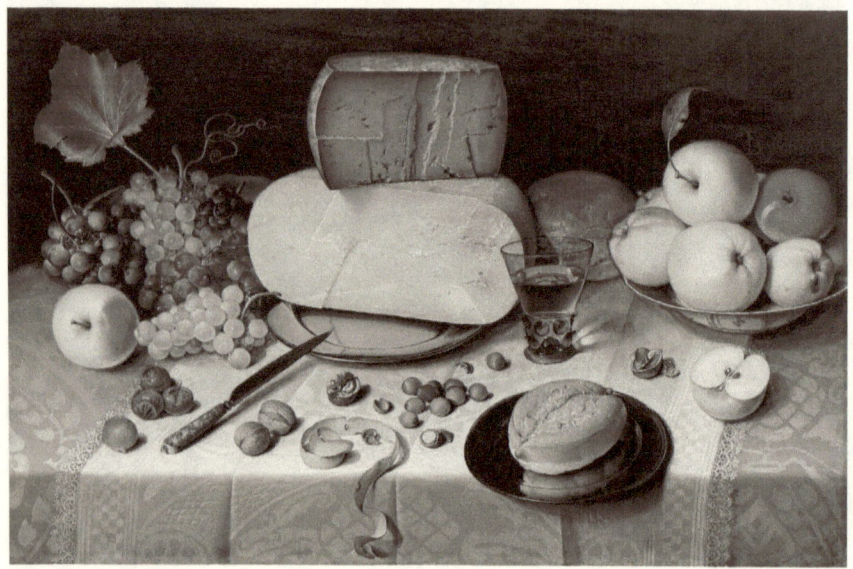

French banquets are the first class of food enjoyment and has an abundance of variety. Even the simplest food will be full of elegance and charm. The French love to test their taste buds. The normal French banquet lasts for five to six hours. They like to sample the food and go about it slowly. There are various courses.

The first course is *l'aperitif*, where the host treats the guests to champagne or cocktail or other drinks they like. Light appetizers will be served to stimulate their appetite before meals. The host thanks the guests for making it to the banquet. Guests are treated with various sumptuous appetizers during the course. They include both hot and cold appetizers. You can sample the cold beef carpaccio and salmon mousse first, then move to hot sole fillet terrine and cheese soufflé. The main course varies from region to region. It lines up with spreads, salad, rice, and pasta. There are many kinds of meat, like chicken, and seafood, like fish, crabs, or lobster. You can pair the foods with wine and drinks. Cheese, a cheese board is lined with a variety of chesses on one side and fruits, nuts, and baguette bread on the other side with wines. Dessert—mostly light desserts such as chocolate mousse, profiteroles, and apple tarts are served. Coffee—most kinds of coffee are served with chocolate truffle or dark chocolate because they boost the taste of coffee. Guest can also choose tea. Dessert is served if it marks the end of the banquet. Mostly strong alcohols like brandy, whisky, or cognac are offered.

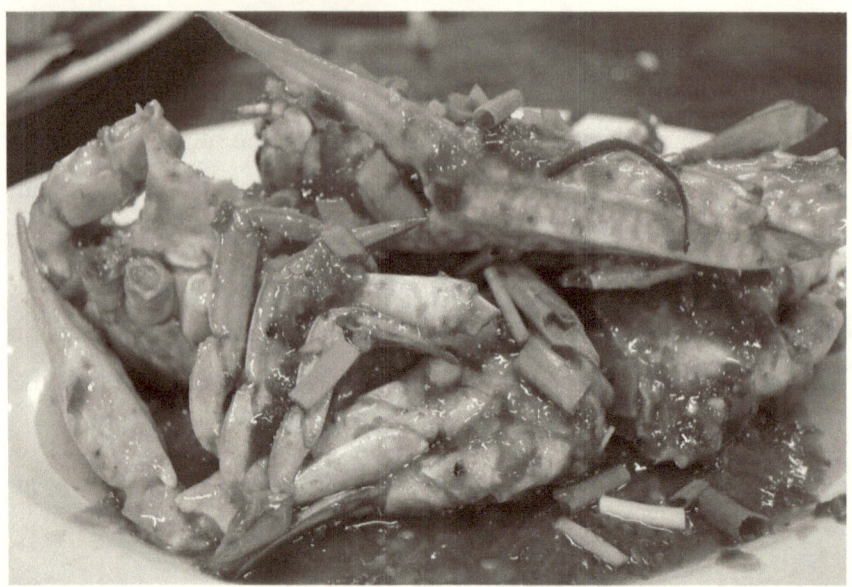

English afternoon tea—mostly served in a tearoom. The first serve is a combination of a choice of sandwiches, cake, cones. A beautiful teapot and a cup of flower tea are then served. The atmosphere is quiet, and people can chat with one another. Sometimes, there are events, like fashion show will be held to entertain the customers.

Cocktail party—it's the reception that the host holds for the guests to socialize before the event starts. Cocktails will be served with some appetizers. It will be boring if you cannot talk to people. Only those who go around and exchange name cards will have fun. Others stay there smiling, pretending they like the dinner. A companion who goes with you will make you happier.

Crab feed—usually, it's a fundraising event. Buy a ticket first, and the sponsorship will cost more. The event opens with a cash bar, a fantastic silent auction, dessert auction, and great company. An all-you-can-eat salad, pasta, bread, and crab buffet will be served, and you can finish the evening with dance music provided by the DJ. There may be a best table decoration contest. Doors open at noon for people to go in and decorate the table. The event will be promoted through fliers. An event goal must be set. Then you decide how many attendants there should be. Describe the location—where it is, what amenities it provides? The date set for gathering is usually on a Sunday. How many crabs should be ordered? Many find three pounds per person is good. Crab is ordered as a whole cooked crab.

In these occasions, some provide beer. Raffles will promote the events. If it is an annual event, members and community leaders look forward to it, and it becomes more successful each year. Referrals of customers mean it is successful.

Wedding dinner—an invitation card will be sent out to make sure you know how many guests will go to your wedding dinner. Sometimes, you will find some of the guests you don't know. Later, you may know them by the introduction of your parents. It may be held in hotel or a big restaurant. A cocktail reception may be held first. Some have forms of amusement, like playing cards. At the dinner, an address will be made by the parents to introduce the new couples. Dinner will begin. The menu may be several courses. The first one is salad, then the main course, and the last is dessert. People from different ethnic may have more than ten courses.

Ten courses of chicken, fish, vegetables, and meats
Soup
Dessert

At the end of the dinner, the host will bid farewell to the guests. Some will give each guest a present to bless each other. It may be a great cost for some people, but they think they must spend the money. A wedding is a once-in-a-lifetime event. They must celebrate it.

White House State Dinner— US National Dinner

President Barack Obama and First Lady Michelle Obama host a state dinner in honor of French President Francois Hollande. It will be a night filled with glamour, celebrity, power, the best food, fine wines and high class entertainment. Guests will be invited to the dinner event.

The menu

The menu will reflect the best of American cuisine. In keeping with that theme, the ingredients for each course will have a local flair: Caviar, farmed from the estuaries of Illinois; a dozen varieties of potatoes, from New York, Caliornia; dry-aged rib eye beef, from a family owned farm in Colorado; chocolate from Hawaii; tangerines from Florida; and blue cheese and maple syrup from Vermont.

First Course

American Osetra Caviar
Fingerling Potato Veloute, Quail Eggs, Crisped Chive Potatoes

Second Course

The White Garden Salad
Petite Mixed Radish, Baby Carrot, Merlot Lettuce
Red Wine Vineigrette

Main Course

Dry aged Rib-Eye Beef
Japer Hill Farm Blue Cheese, Charred Shallots Oyster
Mushrooms, Braised Chard

Dessert

Hawaiian Chocolate- Malted Ganache
Vanilla Ice Cream and Tangerines

The Wine List

Morlet "La Proportion Doree" 2011
Napa Valley, California
Chester –Kidder Ked Blend 2009
Columbia Valley, Washington
Thibaut-Jannison: Blane de Chardonnay"
Monticello, Virginia

The Entertainment

The entertainment will be American R&B singer, Mary J. Blige, will give an after-dinner serenade.

The Décor

The theme of the dinner's décor was inspired by the shared history and long standing friendship between the United States and France, which will showcase several French pieces, including an exquisite 14-foot mirrored plateau table crafted by French artist Deniere et Matelin and chosen by President James Monroe in 1817.

The 300 guests will dine in pavilion tent on the White House South Lawn dotted with French-inspired bouquets and vines arranged by White House Chief Floral Designer Laura Dowling.

The Guest List

The official guest list have a mix of politicians, celebrities and members of the country's business elite.

The French President Francois Hollande will be invited to the dining room. The United States President, Barack Obama will address first and dinner will begin. After-dinner entertainment will be performed by the singer Mary J. Blige. Guest can chat around. Finally, the dinner ended with cheers.

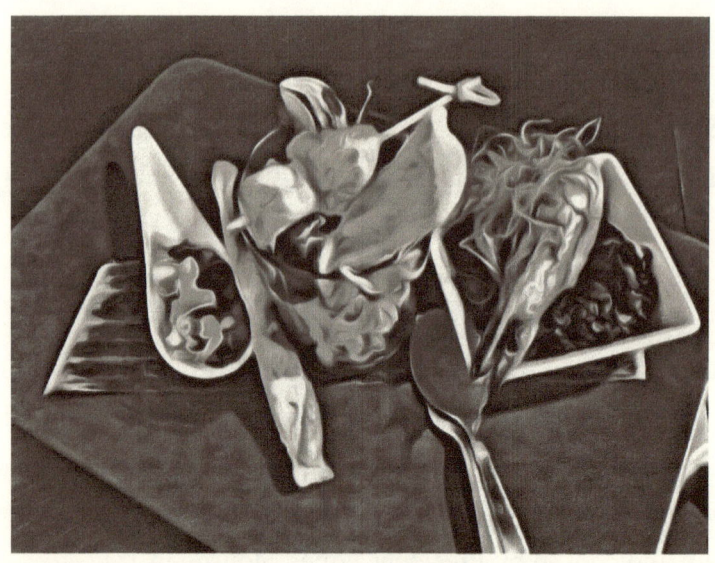

The Most Famous Banquet—the Imperial Feast, Manchurian Han Banquet

It's the most elaborate meal on earth. It's the imperial feast. It takes many chefs three months travelling to different provinces to gather all materials, then use three weeks to prepare, and finally, three days to try and to test all the 108 dishes. In addition, there are 88 small dishes with their 88 different condiments. The food may come from the sky, the land, and the sea. Quality is the selection criterion. The tableware is fine porcelain and silverware. Palace music will be played with the feast. Waiters and waitresses wear beautiful palace gowns. The imperial feast will last for three days and have six separate banquets. Now, the content, etiquette, customs, and formalities are gradually simplified and the number of dishes reduced. After guests are seated, a big red robe tea will be served. Then the banquet will be started with apples and oranges served with seeds and nuts. Cold dish will be served with wine. Wine and drinks will be refilled throughout the feast. The dish ranges from ordinary, such as rice, dumplings,

Peking duck, roast chicken rabbit with hot pepper, white fungus with pigeon eggs; to the unusual, such as bear paws; and off-putting, brains of living monkeys. At the end of the feast, a small silver tray of toothpicks, betel nut, and round cardamom kernels are provided. A wet towel will be used for cleaning your mouth and face. It's the enjoyment of food and event activities.

Now, people will not try this expensive banquet. It may cost over US $10,000. It needs too many cooks and servers. Rooms are needed for them to rest. Many kinds of food are not served, and etiquette is not always strictly followed. Nowadays, the menu will be modified to a smaller number of courses, and the price is cheaper. It fits many restaurants and customers. Housewives can learn the food by observation and ask the chef of the restaurant. The best of the mini Man Han feast can be applied to the family dinner.

We Like Our Home Food

There are plenty of foods. Some need to cook, some are semi-ready-made, some are ready to eat. The food service has the operational concept that figures out the atmosphere, decor, type of service, price structure, and menu planning. We still like our home food. The food from the restaurant is more expensive, takes more time, and requires more management.

Our home food is the best dining experience. The food, the cooking, and eating are what we like most. It can be a normal meal, a family meal, potluck, barbecue, hot pot, a family banquet, Thanksgiving, Christmas, and New Year's dinner.

Every day, we have to plan the meal first. There are three normal meals and one snack meal. What food do we have to prepare? Can they be brought from the nearby supermarket? The recipe will be modified because some don't like fish while some don't eat pork. Sometimes they like to make some new food. So they follow the new recipe or design a new recipe. Sometimes, they find out the result is a mess. The recipe is not detailed enough. Lucky, an angel shows up to help them.

Usually, they, mainly females, learn from the mother or their friends. First they learn how to peel the cucumber or wash the vegetable. Then in cutting the meat, the cut should be diagonal with the line of meats. Next is cooking, which may done by frying, steaming, boiling. They also have to learn the matching of food. Lamb and watermelon will hurt the air duct. Crab stomach will cause abdominal pain, onion and honey will hurt the eyes, potato and banana will hurt facial skin, tofu and honey will cause deafness.

There are no real recipes for cooking. Usually, the recipe will not be detailed. It is by experience. No people will measure the quantity of food. By experience, they know how much food they need for this meal. If more people like this dish, then they will make more. The equipment will be limited to the kitchen facilities, such as microwaves, stoves. Sanitation is based on common sense. The way of preparing food is such that you make sure it doesn't cause sickness and people will be healthy. Damaged canned food will be thrown away, or people will remind you it is not safe. Portions of damaged food with molds will be cut away. They learn to prepare pantry products like appetizers, salads, sandwiches and beverages like coffee and tea. They also prepare stocks, soup, and sauces. Later, it is fruits and vegetables. Finally, it is the meat, poultry, and seafood. They learn one by one with the guidance of their mothers until they can make it exactly like the one made by their mothers. When they can make a meal on their own, it is very happy. Male are not born to be cooks. They just want to ease their hunger. They prefer to go out to eat.

When their cooking becomes more skillful, they will try to modify the dish and design a new dish. They boil the water and add the spaghetti. The spaghetti is ready by testing its tenderness, if it's al dente or if it can break easily. The spaghetti is poured into a filtering bowl and rinsed. Oil is then added in the pan. Then you add spaghetti sauce with mushroom stripes, carrot stripes, and meatballs. The sauce mixture turns into an amazing appearance, the sweet smell is strong. It can stir your appetite. The taste is delicious. The noodle is soft and the sauce is like a great seasoning. Just after a while, it is finished. It is a happy time. The test is simple: just see how much leftover food there is in the plate. Food is simple, but cooking is great. Even a simple food can be a great dish. It will soon make them a good cook.

Men are different. They want to make the preparation of food as simple as putting it in the microwave. Cooking is too casual. The chicken is cut into pieces, but some parts of it have bones while some have no bones. What kind of oil to use, whether to season before or after cooking are the points of argument. Usually, it ends up by saying "I like it, this is good way of cooking" or running away. Frying fish, it depends on the fire (high, medium, or low) or the temperature of cooking. First, heat the oil, then put the fish in the pan. This way, the fish will not stick to the pan if it is not a nonstick pan. The heat should be high, then set to medium. But the men can never predict the time to switch the heat.

Spreading the salt on the body of the fish can eliminate its odor and stabilize the oil temperature. The men are always lazy to do it. Only touching the hot pan, they will keep silent and never yell when it is painful. This dish only results in a mother's comment of the food being bad dish. A soup of cucumber is a good soup. After peeling, cut the cucumber into four pieces. Then cut it into a small piece. One bowl of soup of one cucumber can make it delicious. It is like pouring water make it taste like water. The result is next time, you make a water soup. Don't waste time preparing the cucumber.

Sometimes, they don't know how to cook the food like New York steak, tomato soup. They will ask those friends who know how to cook and teach them. The last choice is to go to a restaurant and buy food to-go. They can order catering if they want to.

There are different table services, American style, French style. Usually, a family meal is freestyle. You can sit together or buffet-style. Soon, they can find out a way to accommodate everybody. Sometimes they will have Thanksgiving, Christmas, and New Year's dinner. Turkey will be included. The standard is salad, soup, mash potato, bread, turkey, and cake. It will be table-style, eating and talking at the same time. Christmas can have exchanging gift activities. Once in a while, a picnic is fun. The food may be sandwich, fruit, salad, or barbecue. The most important thing is to have a suburban view, a sea view, a mountain view, or a plateau view. It can make you have a spiritual mind.

Barbecuing is a fun activity. It can be held in the backyard or outdoors. Doing it outdoors is fun, but backyard barbecue is convenient. A long time ago, people hunted animals. They cut them into pieces or roast them whole. They set a fire and poked the animal with a branch and roasted the animal under the fire. Nowadays, it is for pleasure. We have fast-burning charcoal or gas. Then, we have hot dog, meat sliced already. We cook it with a large fork or tongs to turn it side to side. All kinds of sauce like ketchup, mustard, seasonings are on the dining table.

Eating is freestyle. Of course, with some food, you need some eating skill. If you eat the stomach of a crab, later you will have abdominal pain. The teapot used after crab feed is for washing hands, not for drinking. Meat needs to be cooked in the appropriate temperature. Vegetables must be washed although this will wash away the vitamin. Washing vegetables is to wash away the organic pesticide and the dirt.

Eating is a real enjoyment. That's why they like home food. It's a great dining experience. No matter if it's a formal family gathering or people are a little hungry, have no appetite, and or in a bad mood, they will find something they like to eat. Every day, we need two thousand calories for energy. It's divided into three meals. When we don't have energy, the energy will be produced from the liver. We feel hungry. No appetite, we have to stimulate our appetite. No mood, we need to relax, maybe sleep, to feel good. The worry of employment or living needs to be set aside until we feel better. Comfort food like ice cream or chocolate can be used. A normal condition means we can have common food or great food. It is not only for hunger but also for its flavor for the enjoyment of life.

Conclusion

Food services have operational concept for the customers. They consider the kind of food, types of food service, decor, menu, atmosphere, and other unique features. They base it on large market research. They fit all types or a specific type of customers.

Ethnic food services fit people's appetites and their culture. They know the dining culture already. But more people prefer their family dining. Sometimes, ethnic food services can replace it. Individuals and family are familiar with the dining experience already. Besides hunger pushing that you can eat anything, it is also by appetite. It makes the food acceptable to the taste of the individual. The sense, color, and taste are already accepted.

Of course, it is affected by social and cultural effects. A stronger sense of family causes the people to return to family dining. It begins with from childhood to adulthood and travels worldwide in the contact of others. Culture determines food patterns or habits. Food culture differs around the world, and one may oppose the other, like eating insect food. A family will develop its own characteristic food pattern, and individuals may have preferences for food. They learn what is acceptable or not from the family. Religious people have food laws to follow, like the Muslims, who don't eat pork.

Individuals can enjoy the choice of food that a food service cannot predict. Besides being familiar with family food, they can modify by choosing the food they like or dislike.

Sample of Home Food

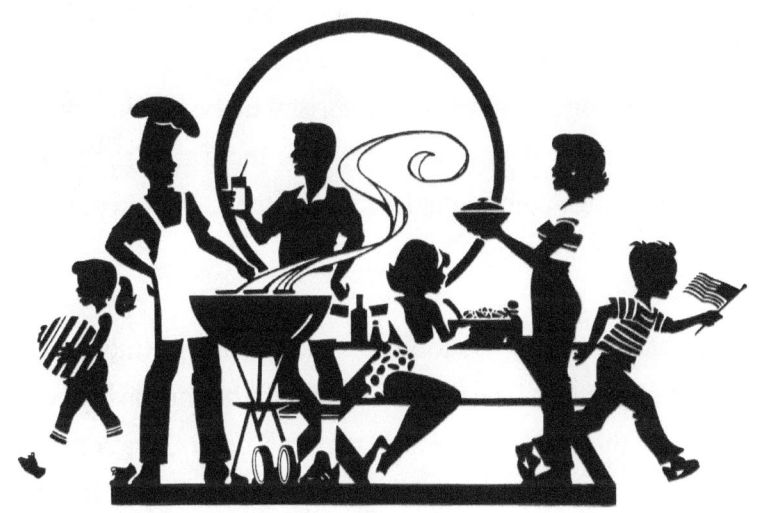

Shrimp, one pound/person

Three or four crabs

Red, white wine, soda, juice

Cocktail sauce or soy sauce with ginger

Coffee and tea

It is fun for family or social gatherings. Put on the tables all the utensils, crab tools, drinks, and sauces. When the food is ready, then, everybody can enjoy the food. The dining experience should be the same as what we have experienced before. It has been proven and tested to be entertaining for many years already. Now, this may be modified a little to make it perfect.

Boil a large bowl of water so that it can cover all the food. Put only a little seasoning of salt because we want to taste the natural seasoning of the crabs and shrimps. When the water is boiling, put the shrimps and crabs into it one by one. Put the shrimp in the bowl, making sure the water can cover all the shrimp. When the water is reboiled and the shrimps change color completely, take them out and put them on the large plate and serve.

When the friends enjoy the food, put more shrimps into the boiling water. The cooking will be the same until all the shrimps are cooked. Or you cook the crab first. When the crab colors, that of the shell and of the meat, are all changed completely, take it out. It may take ten minutes. Then remove the lungs and the stomach, especially the stomach, since it will hurt your stomach. You can remove it before or after cooking. It's better to cut it into four pieces. The shrimp and the crab can be cooked at any sequence; make sure the supply of food is continuous. When the guests are half-full, the cooking may be slowed down so that they have more time to digest the food.

You can use the crab tool to take out the meat for eating. You can also chew the whole leg, but beware of the shell; that may hurt your mouth. Shrimp is easy; just take off the shell and the head. Then, enjoy the shrimp meat. The sauce can be cocktail sauce, or Asians use soy sauce with ginger. Ginger can remove any bad odor. That will be more healthy. Wine, beer, soda will be served. You can talk when you enjoy the food, usually when you are half-full. Then, you may eat slowly. This can help your digestion. At last, coffee and tea will help you clear your stomach. You can go on talking while someone clears the table. When you feel tired, then you can finish the party.

Different people of the world enjoy the same seafood, but the cooking method and eating style are different. Some like spicy or strongly seasoned food. You can also use a ready-made seafood seasoning from the grocery store. The natural taste of the seafood will be the best. Later, you can season it according to your personal preference. The dining experience is what you like. It has been tested for many years. Almost everything is the same.

The atmosphere is good. Service is DIY. It is entertaining. You can talk or eat any way you like. Nobody will stare at you when you eat noisily. No one from the next table and is watching a football game and making it noisy will bother you. If you ask them to keep quiet, they may not care about you. It's the problem of restaurant management. They can control the staff, but they cannot control the customers. Some customers like this while some customers like that. If there are conflicts, the customers may not listen to your solution. That's why some restaurants have a banquet room to separate the customers' groups.

Home food atmosphere is perfect. Any complaint can be resolved by saying a few words. You can choose to go to watch TV while you eat. The most important thing is they know your eating habit. If you don't like spicy food, a separate plate of food will be served for you.

It is entertaining, healthy, comfortable and delicious food for a family gathering. Homeland food is the best. It has been tested for many years already and will go prove to be the best.

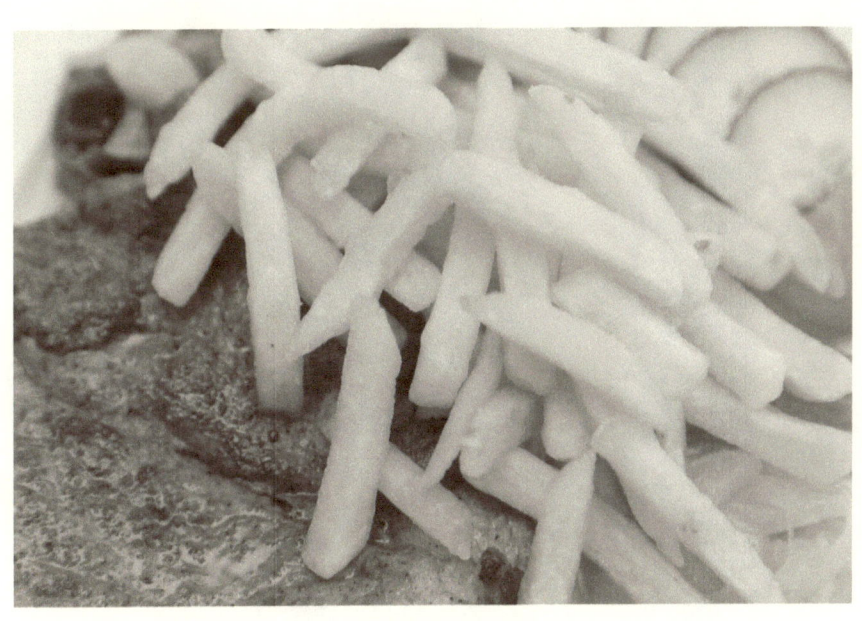

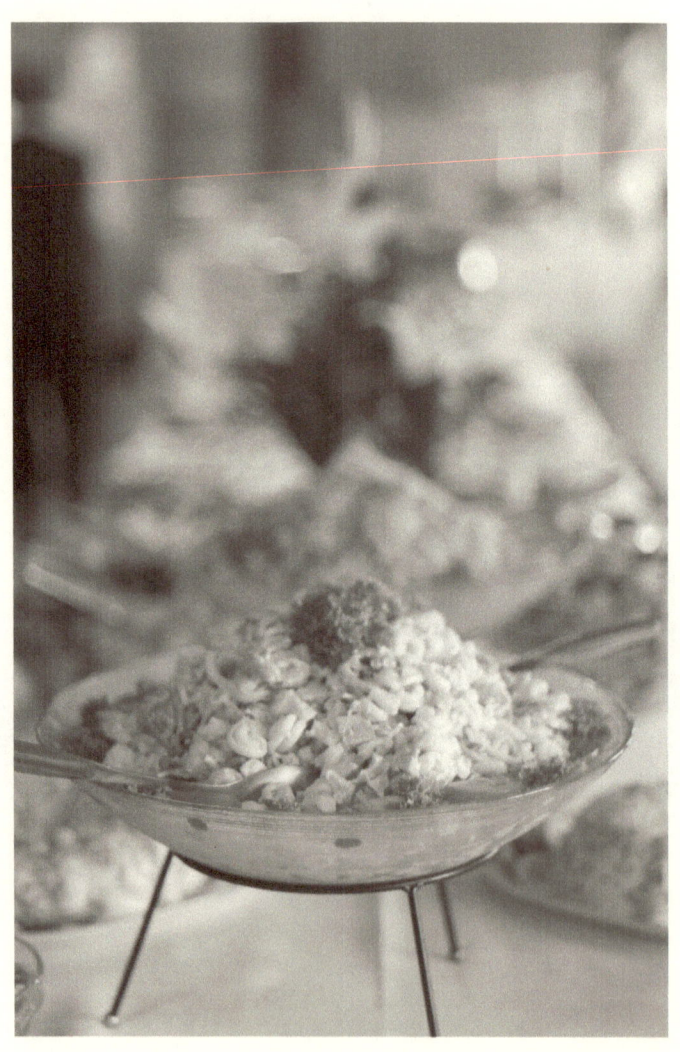